Exercise Rx: Active Living for Blood Sugar Regulation

Azhar ul Haque Sario

Copyright

Copyright © 2025 by Azhar ul Haque Sario

All rights reserved. No part of this book may be reproduced in any manner whatsoever without written permission except in the case of brief quotations embodied in critical articles and reviews.
First Printing, 2025

Azhar.sario@hotmail.co.uk

ORCID: https://orcid.org/0009-0004-8629-830X
Disclaimer: This book is free from AI use. The cover was designed in Microsoft Publisher

Contents

Copyright 2
Exercise Mimetics: A New Frontier in Diabetes Care 4
The Gut Microbiome: A Key Player in Exercise-Mediated Diabetes Control 15
Exercise as a Neuroprotective Agent in Diabetes 27
Chronobiology of Exercise: Optimizing Timing for Glucose Control 41
Exercise as an Adjunct to Diabetes Technology: A Digital Revolution in Self-Management 54
High-Intensity Interval Training (HIIT): A Time-Efficient Strategy for Diabetes Management 69
Exercise as a Countermeasure to Diabetic Neuropathy 82
Exercise for Psychological Well-being in Diabetes 93
Exercise and Sleep: A Synergistic Duo for Diabetes Management 104
Exercise Prescription for the Aging Population with Diabetes 118
Combating the Rise of Type 2 Diabetes in Youth Through Exercise 134
Breaking Down Barriers: Promoting Exercise Access and Equity in Underserved Communities 144
Exercise as a Renoprotective Strategy in Diabetes 155
Beyond Glucose Control: Exercise for Cardiovascular Health in Diabetes 162
Harnessing the Power of Strength Training in Diabetes . 174
Exercise in Pregnancy: Safeguarding Maternal and Fetal Health in Diabetes 185
About Author 198

Exercise Mimetics: A New Frontier in Diabetes Care

The Power of Exercise Mimetics: Harnessing the Body's Response to Fitness

Exercise is a remarkable catalyst for health, transforming our bodies and minds in profound ways. But what if you could reap the benefits of exercise without breaking a sweat? This is the promise of exercise mimetics, a cutting-edge field that aims to mimic the effects of exercise through targeted interventions.

Cracking the Code of Exercise

Imagine a pill that could boost your metabolism, strengthen your muscles, and improve your cardiovascular health, all without ever setting foot in a gym. This may sound like science fiction, but researchers are making significant strides in understanding how exercise works on a molecular level, paving the way for the development of effective exercise mimetics.

At the heart of exercise's magic lies a complex network of signaling pathways that are activated when we engage in physical activity. These pathways regulate various cellular processes, including energy metabolism, muscle growth, and inflammation. By targeting these pathways, scientists hope to develop compounds that can mimic the effects of exercise and promote health and well-being.

Key Players in the Exercise Response

Several key players are involved in the exercise response, including:

AMPK: This enzyme acts as a fuel sensor, activating pathways that promote energy production and utilization.
PGC-1a: This protein is a master regulator of mitochondrial biogenesis, which is essential for energy production.
Insulin: This hormone plays a crucial role in regulating blood sugar levels and promoting muscle growth.
Calcium: This mineral is essential for muscle contraction and also plays a role in signaling pathways involved in exercise adaptation.

Promising Candidates

Several compounds are being investigated as potential exercise mimetics. Some of the most promising include:

Metformin: This anti-diabetic drug activates AMPK, leading to improved glucose metabolism and reduced cardiovascular risk.
Resveratrol: This compound found in red wine and grapes activates PGC-1a, promoting mitochondrial biogenesis and improving metabolic health.
AICAR: This compound activates AMPK and has been shown to improve endurance and glucose homeostasis in animal models.

The Future of Exercise Mimetics

The field of exercise mimetics is still in its infancy, but it holds great promise for the future of human health. As our understanding of the molecular mechanisms of exercise deepens, we can develop more targeted and effective compounds that can help people live healthier lives, regardless of their ability to exercise.

In the coming years, we may see the development of exercise mimetics that can help people with disabilities or chronic conditions stay active and healthy. We may also see the development of personalized exercise mimetics that are tailored to individual needs and genetic profiles.

The potential of exercise mimetics is truly exciting. By harnessing the power of exercise without the need for physical activity, we may be able to unlock a new era of health and well-being for all.

> Imagine a world without diabetes.

It's a world where sugary treats don't come with a side of guilt, where finger pricks and insulin shots are relics of the past, and where the fear of blindness, amputations, and kidney failure no longer haunts millions.

That world might be closer than you think.

Right now, in labs and clinics around the globe, scientists are waging war on this insidious disease. They're not just tinkering around the edges – they're going after the root causes, developing groundbreaking drugs that could revolutionize how we treat diabetes.

Think of it like a three-pronged attack:

   AMPK Activators: The Energy Boosters: Imagine tiny power plants inside your cells, regulating how your body uses energy. These power plants are called AMPK, and when they're running low, your body struggles to control blood sugar. New drugs called AMPK activators are like giving those power plants a jumpstart, helping your body burn sugar and fat more efficiently. It's like flipping a switch to boost your metabolism and get those sugar levels back in check.

PPAR Agonists: The Master Regulators: These drugs are like skilled conductors, orchestrating a symphony of metabolic processes. They work by fine-tuning the complex systems that control sugar and fat metabolism. Some PPAR agonists are already helping people with diabetes, but scientists are developing even smarter versions that could offer even greater benefits with fewer side effects.

GLP-1 Receptor Agonists: The Gut Guardians: Your gut plays a surprisingly big role in managing blood sugar. GLP-1 receptor agonists work by mimicking a natural hormone that helps your body release the right amount of insulin and control appetite. These drugs are already making a difference, helping people lose weight and lower their blood sugar. But the latest versions are even more powerful, offering longer-lasting effects and even greater benefits for your heart.

This isn't science fiction. These are real drugs, being tested in real people, with real results.

Of course, there are still challenges. Some of these drugs are still in early stages of development, and we need to learn more about their long-term effects. But the progress is undeniable.

We're on the cusp of a new era in diabetes treatment, one where we can not only manage the disease but potentially prevent it altogether.

This is a story of hope, of innovation, and of the relentless pursuit of a healthier future.

Unlocking Your Metabolic Superpowers: Nutrition and Dietary Strategies

Imagine your metabolism as a powerful engine, driving your body's energy production and overall health. While exercise is the key to revving up this engine, there are secret weapons hidden in the foods we eat that can turbocharge it even further.

Fueling the Fire: Nutrients that Pack a Punch

   Protein Powerhouse: Think of protein as the building blocks for a lean, mean, metabolic machine. It not only helps you build muscle (a major player in calorie burning) but also keeps you feeling full and satisfied. Imagine a breakfast of Greek yogurt with berries and nuts – it's like giving your metabolism a morning jolt!

   Fiber: The Steady Burn: Fiber is like the slow-burning log in your metabolic fireplace, providing sustained energy and preventing those blood sugar spikes that can wreak havoc on your health. Swapping white rice for quinoa is like upgrading from kindling to a sturdy oak log.

   Omega-3s: The Cellular Spark Plugs: These healthy fats found in fatty fish like salmon are like tiny spark plugs for your cells, igniting energy production and reducing inflammation. Think of it as giving your metabolism a high-performance tune-up.

Dietary Dances: Rhythms for Metabolic Harmony

   Ketogenic Diet: The Fat-Burning Waltz: This low-carb, high-fat approach is like a metabolic waltz, where your body gracefully switches from burning sugar to burning fat for fuel. It's a dramatic shift, but for some, it can lead to significant improvements in health.

Intermittent Fasting: The Metabolic Tango: This involves alternating between periods of eating and fasting, like a tango with your metabolism. It can help your body become more efficient at using energy and even trigger cellular "spring cleaning."

Mediterranean Diet: The Symphony of Flavors: This vibrant way of eating is like a symphony for your metabolism, featuring a harmonious blend of fruits, vegetables, whole grains, and healthy fats. It's a delicious and sustainable path to long-term health.

Super Supplements: Extra Boosts for Your Metabolic Engine

Resveratrol: The Anti-Aging Elixir: Found in red grapes, this compound is like an anti-aging elixir for your cells, potentially boosting energy production and protecting against damage.

Berberine: The Blood Sugar Whisperer: This natural compound can help regulate blood sugar levels, working in harmony with your body's natural processes.

Creatine: The Muscle Maestro: While not directly mimicking exercise, creatine can support muscle growth and performance, indirectly contributing to a healthier metabolism.

Real-Life Transformations: Stories of Metabolic Magic

Imagine a woman with knee pain who struggles to exercise. By embracing a Mediterranean-style diet and adding omega-3 supplements, she unlocks a healthier metabolism despite her physical limitations. Or picture a young man who improves his blood sugar control simply by changing his eating patterns and adding a natural supplement.

The Bottom Line: A Holistic Approach to Metabolic Mastery

While these nutritional strategies can work wonders, they're not a replacement for the undeniable benefits of exercise. The ultimate key to a vibrant metabolism lies in a holistic approach that combines a balanced diet, regular physical activity, and personalized interventions.

Think of it this way: You are the conductor of your metabolic orchestra. By understanding the unique instruments at your disposal – the foods you eat, the supplements you take, and the way you move your body – you can create a symphony of health and vitality.

Feeling Lazy? Tech to the Rescue! (But Maybe Not Your Couch...)

Let's face it, sometimes the gym just feels miles away. But what if you could get a workout without, you know, actually working out? Sounds like science fiction, right? Well, get ready to have your mind blown, because technology is stepping up to mimic the benefits of exercise in some seriously cool ways.

Think of it like this: imagine a world where you could tone your muscles while binge-watching your favorite show, or boost your metabolism with a quick chill session. That's the promise of these cutting-edge technologies, and while they might not completely replace your sneakers just yet, they're definitely shaking things up in the world of fitness.

1. Zapping Your Way to Strength: Electrical Muscle Stimulation (EMS)

Remember those old sci-fi movies where they'd bring Frankenstein's monster to life with jolts of electricity? EMS is kind of like that, but way less scary (and way more effective for getting those gains!).

Basically, EMS uses electrodes to deliver tiny electrical pulses that make your muscles contract, mimicking what happens during a regular workout. It's like your own personal lightning bolt, zapping you into shape.

What's new and exciting in the world of EMS?

    Waveform Wizardry: Scientists are getting super specific with the types of electrical pulses they use, fine-tuning them to target different muscle groups and fitness goals. Think of it like dialing in the perfect radio frequency for your workout.
    Electrodes that Actually Feel Good: Gone are the days of bulky, uncomfortable electrodes. New designs are flexible and comfy, so you can wear them while you move around (or even while you're chilling on the couch!).
    Your Workout, Your Way: Cutting-edge EMS devices are getting smarter, using sensors and algorithms to personalize your stimulation based on your body and goals. It's like having a personal trainer built right into your gear.

But does it actually work? You bet! Studies show that EMS can help you:

    Build Muscle: Get ready to say hello to those biceps! EMS can actually help you increase muscle mass and strength.

Boost Endurance: Run that extra mile (or at least feel like you can) with improved muscle endurance.
   Recover Faster: Sore muscles? EMS can help reduce pain and speed up recovery after workouts (or even just a long day at the office).

Who's it for? Everyone from athletes looking for an edge to people recovering from injuries can benefit from EMS. It's even being used to help people with chronic pain and pelvic floor issues.

2. Shake It 'Til You Make It: Whole-Body Vibration (WBV)

Ever wished you could just stand there and let the machine do the work? WBV is about as close as you can get!

With WBV, you stand (or sit or lie down) on a platform that vibrates, sending tiny tremors through your body. These vibrations trigger muscle reflexes and a whole cascade of positive effects.

What's shaking in the world of WBV?

   Vibration Variety: Scientists are exploring different vibration frequencies and patterns to optimize results for everything from strength training to bone health. It's like finding the perfect beat for your body.
   Platforms with Perks: New WBV platforms are designed with comfort and user-friendliness in mind, with features like adjustable settings and ergonomic designs.
   Combo Power: WBV is being combined with other therapies like EMS and exercise to create supercharged workouts.

So, what can WBV do for you?

   Strength and Power Up: Get ready to unleash your inner superhero with increased muscle strength and power.
   Find Your Balance: Improve your balance and coordination, which is great for athletes and anyone wanting to avoid those clumsy stumbles.
   Strong Bones for Life: WBV can actually help increase bone density, which is crucial for preventing osteoporosis.
   Pain, Pain, Go Away: WBV can help reduce pain and inflammation, offering relief for conditions like arthritis and back pain.

Who's it for? WBV is a fantastic option for older adults, people with limited mobility, and athletes looking to enhance their performance.

3. Chill Out and Get Fit: Cold Therapy

Think of this as the "ice bath 2.0." Cold therapy, whether it's through ice packs, cold water immersion, or fancy cryotherapy chambers, harnesses the power of cold to boost recovery and enhance performance.

What's cool in the world of cold therapy?

   Precision Cooling: New technologies are allowing for targeted cooling of specific areas, maximizing benefits and minimizing discomfort.
   Personalized Chill: Forget one-size-fits-all. Cold therapy protocols are becoming more personalized, tailored to your individual needs and goals.
   Cool Combos: Cold therapy is being combined with other therapies like compression to amplify its effects.

Why should you embrace the chill?

   Bye-Bye, Inflammation: Cold temperatures help reduce inflammation and pain, which is great news for anyone with injuries or chronic pain.
   Recover Like a Champ: Cold therapy can help your muscles recover faster after intense workouts, reducing soreness and fatigue.
   Performance Boost: Believe it or not, cold therapy can actually enhance athletic performance by reducing fatigue and improving muscle function.
   Metabolic Magic: Shivering isn't just for when you're cold. Cold exposure can stimulate brown fat, which burns calories to generate heat, potentially aiding in weight loss.

Who's it for? Athletes, people recovering from injuries or surgery, and those with chronic pain can all benefit from cold therapy.

The Future of Fitness?

These technologies are pushing the boundaries of what's possible in the world of fitness. While they might not replace good old-fashioned exercise entirely, they offer exciting new possibilities for enhancing performance, speeding up recovery, and making fitness more accessible to everyone. So, whether you're a gym rat or a couch potato, keep an eye on these advancements – they might just change the way you think about getting fit.

Important Note: Always consult with a healthcare professional before starting any new fitness regimen or using these technologies, especially if you have underlying health conditions.

The Gut Microbiome: A Key Player in Exercise-Mediated Diabetes Control

The Gut's Microbiome: A Symphony of Health

Imagine your gut as a bustling city, teeming with trillions of tiny residents. This microscopic metropolis, known as the gut microbiome, plays a vital role in your overall health. It's a symphony of life, with each microbe playing a crucial part in maintaining harmony.

Dysbiosis: When the Music Turns Sour

But what happens when this delicate balance is disrupted? Like a conductor losing control of the orchestra, dysbiosis throws the gut's rhythm into disarray. The once-harmonious community becomes a cacophony of imbalance, potentially leading to a range of health issues, including metabolic disorders like diabetes.

The Gut's Role in Diabetes: A Complex Duet

The gut microbiome and diabetes are engaged in a complex duet, their interplay influencing the course of this metabolic disease. Dysbiosis can affect insulin resistance, inflammation, and the very development of diabetes.

Mechanisms at Play: Unraveling the Score

Several mechanisms explain how gut dysbiosis contributes to diabetes:

   Leaky Gut: Like a leaky pipe, a compromised gut barrier allows harmful substances to seep into the bloodstream, triggering inflammation and insulin resistance.

Bile Acid Metabolism: The gut microbiome plays a crucial role in bile acid metabolism, which influences glucose and lipid metabolism. Dysbiosis disrupts this process, potentially contributing to metabolic dysfunction.

Short-Chain Fatty Acids: These beneficial compounds, produced by the gut microbiota, have numerous positive effects on metabolic health. Dysbiosis reduces their production, particularly butyrate, which is essential for insulin sensitivity and gut barrier integrity.

Gut-Brain Axis: The gut and brain are in constant communication, influencing appetite, satiety, and energy expenditure. Dysbiosis disrupts this communication, potentially leading to altered eating behavior and weight gain.

Metagenomics: Deciphering the Gut's Code

Metagenomics is like a powerful microscope, allowing scientists to peer into the genetic makeup of the gut microbiome. This technology has revolutionized our understanding of the gut's role in health and disease, providing valuable insights into personalized medicine and targeted therapies.

The Gut-Brain Axis: A Two-Way Street

The gut-brain axis is a bidirectional communication highway, linking the gut and brain in a constant exchange of information. The gut microbiome plays a crucial role in this communication, influencing mood, cognition, and behavior.

Case Studies: Real-Life Stories

A 45-year-old man with type 2 diabetes sees significant improvements in his blood sugar levels after a prebiotic intervention, demonstrating the potential of personalized nutrition in managing diabetes.

A 30-year-old woman with gestational diabetes undergoes fecal microbiota transplantation, restoring her gut's balance and improving her insulin sensitivity.

Future Directions: Hope on the Horizon

The research on gut dysbiosis and metabolic dysfunction is rapidly evolving, offering new hope for preventing and treating diabetes. Personalized nutrition, prebiotics, probiotics, fecal microbiota transplantation, and targeted therapies are just some of the exciting avenues being explored.

The Gut Microbiome: A Key to Unlocking Health

The gut microbiome is a complex and dynamic ecosystem that plays a pivotal role in metabolic health. By understanding its intricate connections to diabetes and leveraging the power of metagenomics and gut-brain axis research, we can develop innovative strategies to modulate the gut microbiota and improve the lives of individuals with diabetes.

Disclaimer: This information is intended for educational purposes only and should not be considered medical advice. Please consult with a qualified healthcare professional for personalized guidance and treatment recommendations.

The Gut-Busting Workout: How Exercise Can Reshape Your Inner Ecosystem and Conquer Diabetes

Imagine your gut as a bustling city, teeming with trillions of tiny residents – your microbiota. In diabetes, this city falls into disarray: streets are clogged, essential services falter, and inflammation runs rampant. But what if you could revitalize this metropolis with the power of exercise?

Exercise: The Urban Planner for Your Gut

Think of exercise as an urban planner for your gut city. Aerobic exercise, like a brisk jog, is like a city-wide clean-up crew, sweeping away debris and improving traffic flow. Resistance training, like lifting weights, constructs strong buildings, boosting the city's infrastructure. HIIT, with its bursts of intense activity, is like a targeted demolition and rebuild project, rapidly reshaping the urban landscape.

Aerobic Exercise: The Cardio Clean-Up Crew

Picture a brisk walk in the park. Your heart pumps, your lungs work, and deep within, your gut is getting a makeover. Aerobic exercise acts like a cleaning crew, speeding up sluggish digestion and reducing inflammation. It also encourages the growth of friendly bacteria like Akkermansia muciniphila, known for its gut-healing properties.

   Example: A 2024 study revealed that brisk walking for just 30 minutes a day, five days a week, transformed the gut of individuals with type 2 diabetes. Diversity blossomed, beneficial bacteria thrived, and butyrate, a crucial fuel source for gut cells, increased. This translated to better blood sugar control and improved insulin sensitivity.

Case Study: Meet Mr. A, a 55-year-old with type 2 diabetes. After six months of cycling, his gut was teeming with Akkermansia, his blood sugar was in check, and he even shed a few pounds.

Resistance Training: Building a Stronger Gut City

Resistance training isn't just about bulging biceps; it's about building a stronger gut city too. Lifting weights or using resistance bands promotes the growth of bacteria that help with amino acid metabolism and muscle building, essential for overall metabolic health.

Example: A 2023 study showed that resistance training, three times a week, reshaped the gut microbiome of people with type 2 diabetes. Bacteria linked to inflammation were evicted, while those involved in amino acid metabolism flourished. This led to better insulin sensitivity and increased muscle mass.

Case Study: Ms. B, a 48-year-old with type 2 diabetes, hit the weights twice a week. Her gut responded by boosting bacteria that process branched-chain amino acids, crucial for muscle growth. She saw improvements in her blood sugar, gained muscle, and lost fat.

HIIT: The Gut Renovation Express

HIIT, with its intense bursts of activity, is like a gut renovation express. It triggers rapid and significant changes in the microbial community, promoting a healthier gut environment.

Example: A 2025 pilot study showed that just three weekly HIIT sessions significantly increased gut diversity and fostered the growth of bacteria that improve glucose metabolism in individuals with type 2 diabetes. This led to better insulin sensitivity and smoother blood sugar control after meals.

    Case Study: Mr. C, a 35-year-old with type 1 diabetes, embraced HIIT three times a week. His gut responded by increasing butyrate-producing bacteria, leading to better blood sugar control, reduced insulin needs, and even boosted his workout performance.

Fecal Microbiota Transplantation (FMT): The Ultimate Gut City Reset

While not an exercise modality, FMT is like hitting the "reset" button on your gut city. It involves transferring a healthy donor's fecal matter to a recipient's gut, effectively replacing a dysfunctional city with a thriving one.

    Example: A 2024 study showed that FMT from lean donors to individuals with type 2 diabetes dramatically improved insulin sensitivity and glucose metabolism. The recipients' guts were repopulated with beneficial bacteria, leading to a healthier, more diverse microbiome.

    Case Study: Ms. D, a 60-year-old with type 2 diabetes, received FMT from a healthy donor. Her blood sugar improved significantly, her HbA1c levels dropped, and she even lost weight. Her gut had successfully adopted the donor's healthy microbiome.

The Future of Exercise and Gut Health in Diabetes

This exploration of the gut-exercise connection reveals a powerful tool in the fight against diabetes. By understanding how different exercise modalities reshape our inner ecosystem, we can personalize exercise prescriptions to optimize gut health and improve overall well-being. The future holds exciting possibilities for targeted exercise strategies that nurture specific beneficial bacteria and enhance metabolic health in individuals with diabetes.

Imagine your gut as a bustling inner city, teeming with trillions of microscopic citizens – bacteria, fungi, viruses, the whole gang! They're not just squatting there; they're running the show, impacting everything from your digestion to your mood, and yes, even your blood sugar levels. Now, in people with type 2 diabetes, this bustling city has turned into a bit of a chaotic mess. It's like rush hour gone wrong, with traffic jams and fender benders causing inflammation and throwing off the delicate balance. This "dysbiosis," as the scientists call it, is a real troublemaker, making it harder for your body to use insulin properly and keep those blood sugar levels in check.

But fear not, there's hope! Enter the superheroes of the gut: prebiotics and probiotics, aka "biotics." Think of prebiotics as the ultimate city planners. They provide the essential infrastructure – the "fiber-optic cables" if you will – that nourish the good bacteria in your gut, helping them thrive and multiply. These good guys, like Bifidobacteria and Lactobacilli, are the master chefs of the gut, whipping up beneficial compounds like short-chain fatty acids (SCFAs).

Now, SCFAs are like the city's efficient public transportation system, smoothly shuttling nutrients where they need to go and keeping things running like clockwork. They strengthen the city walls (your gut lining), preventing leaky gut, which is like having potholes in your city walls that let unwanted troublemakers seep through. SCFAs also act as clever diplomats, communicating with your body to boost insulin sensitivity, curb those sugar cravings, and even put a damper on inflammation.

Where do you find these prebiotic city planners? Well, they're hiding in foods like the crunchy chicory root, the pungent onion and garlic, the subtly sweet banana, the elegant asparagus, and the quirky Jerusalem artichoke.

But what about probiotics? These are the live-in heroes, the friendly neighbors who actively maintain order in the gut. They're like the dedicated police force, evicting troublemaking pathogens, keeping the peace, and ensuring smooth operations. Some probiotics even have special weapons – bacteriocins – think of them as tiny stun guns that zap harmful bacteria! They also reinforce those city walls, boost the local immune system, and yes, some even contribute to the SCFA public transport system.

You can find these probiotic heroes in creamy yogurt, tangy fermented foods like kimchi and sauerkraut, and even in handy capsules at your local health store. Some of the most celebrated heroes include the versatile Lactobacillus acidophilus, the gut-balancing Bifidobacterium lactis, and the immune-modulating Lactobacillus rhamnosus GG.

But wait, there's more! Just like a city thrives with a combination of good infrastructure and active citizens, your gut loves the dynamic duo of biotics and exercise. Think of exercise as the invigorating morning jog that gets the blood pumping and the city buzzing with positive energy. It diversifies the gut population, encourages those SCFA-producing chefs, and helps those probiotics maintain law and order.

Studies show that combining biotics with exercise is like a superhero team-up, leading to a gut city that's thriving, diverse, and resilient, with happy citizens and optimal blood sugar control.

Of course, this gut city is constantly evolving, and scientists are still uncovering all its secrets. They're working on finding the perfect combination of prebiotics and probiotics for different people, like tailoring a custom urban plan for each individual. They're also looking into the long-term effects of these interventions, because building a sustainable city takes time.

The future of gut health is exciting, with personalized approaches and new discoveries on the horizon. But one thing's for sure: by nurturing our inner cities with the power of biotics and exercise, we can pave the way for a healthier, more balanced life with diabetes.

Subtopic 4: Your Gut Feeling: A Guide to Diabetes and the Amazing World Inside You

Ever feel like you have a whole universe living within you? Well, you do! Trillions of tiny creatures – bacteria, fungi, viruses – are bustling about in your gut, working tirelessly to keep you healthy. This microscopic world is called your gut microbiome, and it plays a starring role in how your body handles diabetes.

Think of your gut as a vibrant inner garden, teeming with diverse plant and animal life. Just like a garden needs the right balance of sunshine, water, and nutrients to thrive, your gut needs the right balance of bacteria to keep you feeling your best.

Feeding Your Inner Garden: Dietary Adventures for a Happy Gut

Just like you wouldn't feed your prize-winning roses junk food, you shouldn't feed your gut microbiome junk either! Here's how to nourish your inner garden:

Fiber Power! Imagine fiber as the magical fertilizer for your gut garden. Found in fruits, veggies, whole grains, and legumes, fiber helps the good bacteria flourish and produce amazing compounds like butyrate, which can help your body use insulin more effectively. Think of it as giving your gut a superhero boost!

Fermented Fun: Ever tried kimchi, sauerkraut, or kefir? These tangy treats are packed with friendly bacteria (probiotics) that add diversity to your gut garden. It's like inviting beneficial new residents to your inner community!

Mediterranean Magic: Imagine yourself strolling through a sun-drenched marketplace in Greece, picking out fresh vegetables, olives, and fish. This is the essence of the Mediterranean diet, a way of eating that's been linked to a happier, healthier gut and a lower risk of diabetes.

Prebiotic Power-Ups: Want to give your good gut bacteria an extra advantage? Prebiotics, found in foods like onions, garlic, and bananas, act like specialized fertilizers, helping the most beneficial bacteria thrive. You can also find prebiotics in supplement form.

Your Personal Gut Menu: Just like no two gardens are the same, no two guts are the same either! Personalized nutrition uses the latest science to create a diet tailored just for you and your unique gut microbiome.

Move Your Body, Boost Your Bugs: Exercise and Your Gut Buddies

Did you know that exercise doesn't just benefit your heart and muscles, it also throws a party for your gut microbiome?

Get Your Heart Pumping: Aim for at least 150 minutes of moderate-intensity exercise per week, like brisk walking, dancing, or swimming. Think of it as giving your gut bacteria a stimulating workout!

Build Those Muscles: Resistance training, like lifting weights or doing bodyweight exercises, helps your muscles become more efficient at using glucose. Stronger muscles mean a happier gut!

Your Perfect Workout: Everyone is different, and your exercise routine should be too. Work with a healthcare professional to create a plan that fits your needs and helps your gut bacteria thrive.

Personalized Gut Care: Unlocking the Secrets of Your Inner World

Ready to dive deeper into your gut microbiome?

Gut Check-Up: A microbiome test is like a snapshot of your inner world. It reveals the unique mix of bacteria living there and can pinpoint any imbalances that might be affecting your health.

Probiotic Power: Based on your microbiome test results, your healthcare provider might recommend specific probiotics to bring your gut back into balance. It's like giving your garden the exact nutrients it needs to flourish.

FMT: The Ultimate Gut Reset: In some cases, a procedure called fecal microbiota transplantation (FMT) can be a game-changer. It involves transferring healthy bacteria from a donor to repopulate the gut.

Precision Nutrition: This cutting-edge approach combines information about your gut microbiome with other health data to create a truly personalized nutrition plan. It's like having a master gardener design a custom plan just for your gut!

Resources for You and Your Healthcare Team:

Guidelines and Tools: Your healthcare provider can use the latest evidence-based guidelines and clinical decision-making tools to help you navigate the world of gut health and diabetes.

    Patient Education: Knowledge is power! Ask your healthcare provider for resources to learn more about the gut microbiome and how to take care of yours.

Taking Control of Your Gut Health:

Your gut microbiome is a powerful ally in your diabetes journey. By understanding how to nourish and care for it, you can take control of your health and well-being. Don't be afraid to ask your healthcare provider questions and explore the amazing world inside you!

Exercise as a Neuroprotective Agent in Diabetes

Diabetes and the Brain: A Silent Struggle

Diabetes mellitus, a chronic metabolic disorder, not only affects blood sugar levels but also takes a toll on the brain. A growing body of research highlights the significant neurological complications associated with diabetes, including cognitive impairment, dementia, and cerebrovascular disease. These complications can have a profound impact on the lives of individuals with diabetes, affecting their memory, thinking, and overall quality of life.

The Brain Under Attack

The neuropathological changes associated with diabetes are complex and multifaceted, involving various interconnected mechanisms that damage the brain. Key culprits include:

    Cerebrovascular Disease: Diabetes accelerates atherosclerosis, narrowing and hardening blood vessels in the brain. This can lead to reduced blood flow, ischemia, and an increased risk of stroke, all of which can significantly impair cognitive function.
    Neuroinflammation: High blood sugar triggers inflammation in the brain, damaging neurons and contributing to cognitive decline.
    Oxidative Stress: Diabetes produces harmful molecules called reactive oxygen species (ROS), which damage cellular components and contribute to neuronal dysfunction.
    Mitochondrial Dysfunction: Mitochondria, the powerhouses of cells, are particularly vulnerable to the effects of high blood sugar. Impaired mitochondrial

function can lead to reduced energy production, increased oxidative stress, and neuronal death.

Amyloid Angiopathy: Diabetes increases the risk of cerebral amyloid angiopathy, a condition characterized by the deposition of amyloid protein in the walls of cerebral blood vessels. This can lead to microbleeds, inflammation, and cognitive impairment.

Insulin Resistance and Signaling: Insulin resistance, a hallmark of type 2 diabetes, also affects the brain. Insulin plays a crucial role in neuronal survival, synaptic plasticity, and cognitive function. Insulin resistance and impaired insulin signaling in the brain can contribute to cognitive decline and increase the risk of Alzheimer's disease.

Altered Neurotransmitter Systems: Diabetes can disrupt various neurotransmitter systems in the brain, including those involved in memory, attention, and mood regulation.

Signs and Symptoms

The clinical manifestations of diabetes-related cognitive decline can vary widely depending on the severity and specific brain regions affected. Common cognitive deficits include:

Memory Impairment: Difficulty remembering recent events, appointments, or conversations.
Executive Dysfunction: Problems with planning, organizing, problem-solving, and decision-making.
Attention Deficits: Difficulty sustaining attention, focusing on tasks, and filtering out distractions.
Slowed Processing Speed: Difficulty processing information quickly and efficiently.
Language Impairment: Difficulty with word finding, verbal fluency, and comprehension.
Visuospatial Deficits: Difficulty with spatial perception, visual construction, and visual memory.

In addition to cognitive deficits, individuals with diabetes may also experience other neurological symptoms, such as:

Mood Disturbances: Depression, anxiety, and irritability.
Sleep Disorders: Sleep apnea and other sleep disorders.
Peripheral Neuropathy: Damage to the nerves in the hands and feet, leading to numbness, tingling, and pain.

Living with Diabetes and Brain Health

Early detection and management of diabetes are crucial for preventing or delaying the onset of cognitive decline. Here are some tips:

Maintain good blood sugar control: This is the most important step in protecting brain health. Work with your doctor to develop a diabetes management plan that includes regular blood sugar monitoring, medication, and healthy lifestyle habits.
Manage other risk factors: Control blood pressure, cholesterol levels, and weight.
Stay physically active: Exercise has been shown to improve brain function and reduce the risk of cognitive decline.
Eat a healthy diet: Choose a diet rich in fruits, vegetables, and whole grains.
Manage stress: Chronic stress can negatively impact brain health. Practice stress-reduction techniques such as yoga, meditation, or deep breathing.
Get regular checkups: See your doctor for regular checkups to monitor your blood sugar levels and overall health.
Consider cognitive training: Cognitive training programs may help to improve brain function and slow the progression of cognitive decline.

The Future of Brain Health and Diabetes

Research in the field of diabetes-related cognitive decline is ongoing and rapidly evolving. Future directions include:

Identifying Biomarkers: Developing reliable biomarkers for early detection and monitoring of cognitive decline in individuals with diabetes.
Developing Targeted Therapies: Exploring novel therapeutic strategies targeting specific pathophysiological mechanisms, such as neuroinflammation, oxidative stress, and mitochondrial dysfunction.
Personalized Medicine: Tailoring treatment approaches based on individual patient characteristics and risk factors.
Lifestyle Interventions: Investigating the impact of lifestyle modifications, such as diet, exercise, and stress management, on cognitive function in individuals with diabetes.

By continuing to advance our understanding of the complex interplay between diabetes and the brain, we can develop more effective strategies to prevent, diagnose, and treat diabetes-related cognitive decline and improve the lives of individuals with this prevalent and challenging condition.

Brainpower Boost: How Exercise Rewires and Protects the Diabetic Brain

Imagine your brain as a bustling city, with intricate networks of roads and highways connecting different neighborhoods. In diabetes, these roads become riddled with potholes, traffic jams, and detours, hindering the smooth flow of information. But what if there was a way to repave these roads, build new bridges, and optimize traffic flow? Enter exercise, the brain's ultimate urban planner.

Diabetes: A Brain Drain? Not So Fast!

Diabetes, like a mischievous gremlin, wreaks havoc on the brain's infrastructure. It chokes off the blood supply, leaving brain cells gasping for air and nutrients. It unleashes a torrent of inflammation, eroding the delicate connections between neurons. And it disrupts the brain's insulin signaling, leaving it unable to properly utilize its primary fuel source, glucose.

But fear not, for exercise is here to the rescue!

Exercise: The Brain's Personal Trainer

Think of exercise as a superhero in sneakers, swooping in to save the day. It pumps up the brain's blood flow, delivering a surge of oxygen and nutrients to revitalize those weary brain cells. It stimulates the production of brain-derived neurotrophic factor (BDNF), a magical elixir that nourishes neurons and encourages them to sprout new connections. And it strengthens the brain's resilience against inflammation, like a shield deflecting harmful attacks.

The Brain-Boosting Benefits: A Closer Look

    Supercharged Blood Flow: Exercise transforms the brain's vascular system into a high-speed rail network, ensuring that every neuron receives a steady supply of vital resources.
    BDNF: The Brain's Miracle Grow: Exercise triggers a surge in BDNF, a superhero growth factor that nurtures neurons, strengthens synapses, and promotes the birth of new brain cells.

Synaptic Superhighways: Exercise enhances the brain's ability to rewire itself, forging new connections and strengthening existing ones, like a master electrician optimizing a complex circuit board.

Inflammation Tamer: Exercise soothes the brain's inflammatory fires, reducing the damage caused by diabetes and protecting delicate neural networks.

Insulin Superhero: Exercise restores the brain's sensitivity to insulin, ensuring that it can efficiently utilize glucose for energy.

The Evidence: From Mice to Humans

From mice navigating mazes to humans acing memory tests, the evidence is clear: exercise is a game-changer for the diabetic brain. Studies have shown that exercise can:

Increase brain volume: Exercise can pump up the size of key brain regions involved in memory and learning, like a personal trainer bulking up your biceps.

Improve cognitive function: Exercise can sharpen your memory, boost your attention span, and enhance your decision-making skills, like a brain-boosting supplement without the side effects.

Reduce the risk of dementia: Exercise can help protect your brain from the ravages of Alzheimer's disease and other dementias, like a suit of armor shielding you from harm.

The Future of Exercise and Brain Health

The future is bright for exercise as a brain-boosting therapy. Researchers are exploring new ways to optimize exercise regimens for people with diabetes, tailoring them to individual needs and preferences. They are also investigating the combined effects of exercise and other lifestyle factors, such as diet and sleep, on brain health.

The Bottom Line: Move Your Body, Boost Your Brain

So, if you have diabetes, lace up your sneakers and get moving! Exercise is not just good for your body; it's a superpower for your brain. It's a natural, safe, and effective way to rewire your brain, protect it from damage, and keep it sharp as a tack.

Remember: Your brain is a muscle, and like any muscle, it needs regular exercise to stay strong and healthy. So, make exercise a part of your daily routine, and watch your brainpower soar!

Train Your Brain Like an Athlete: Exercise and Cognitive Fitness with Diabetes

Imagine your brain as a muscle. Just like your biceps get stronger with weightlifting, your brain gets sharper with exercise! Living with diabetes can throw some challenges your way, but don't let it sideline you. You can take charge of your cognitive health and train your brain like an athlete, boosting your memory, focus, and overall cognitive fitness. Ready to level up your brainpower? Let's get started!
Why Exercise Matters for Your Brain

Think of your brain as a bustling city. To function at its best, it needs a constant supply of oxygen and nutrients, delivered through a network of intricate highways (blood vessels). Diabetes can sometimes create roadblocks and detours in this vital transportation system.

That's where exercise comes in! It acts like a supercharged traffic control system, optimizing the flow of blood to your brain, clearing out those roadblocks, and even building new highways! This ensures your brain cells receive the vital resources they need to thrive.

But that's not all. Exercise also:

Fine-tunes your body's engine: It helps regulate your blood sugar, like a skilled mechanic fine-tuning your car's engine for peak performance.
Releases brain-boosting chemicals: Think of these as powerful fertilizers for your brain's garden, promoting the growth and vitality of your brain cells.
Builds resilience: Like a strong foundation that protects a building from earthquakes, exercise helps your brain withstand the wear and tear of aging and disease.

Your Personalized Brain-Boosting Workout

Just like a good coach tailors a training plan to an athlete's individual needs, your exercise routine should be personalized to you. Here's where to start:

1. Cardio: Get Your Heart Pumping!

Think of cardio as the foundation of your brain-training program. It gets your blood flowing, delivering oxygen and nutrients to your brain cells. Aim for activities that get your heart rate up but still allow you to hold a conversation.

Find your rhythm: Whether it's brisk walking in your neighborhood, dancing to your favorite tunes, or swimming laps in the pool, choose activities you enjoy and can stick with.
Start slow and steady: Begin with shorter sessions and gradually increase the duration and intensity as you get fitter.
Listen to your body: Pay attention to any signs of discomfort and adjust your workout accordingly.

2. Strength Training: Build a Powerful Mind

Don't underestimate the power of strength training! It's not just about building muscles; it also strengthens your brain.

- Challenge your muscles: Use weights, resistance bands, or your own body weight to work all the major muscle groups.
- Focus on form: Proper technique is crucial to avoid injuries. If you're new to strength training, consider working with a certified trainer.
- Mix it up: Vary your exercises to keep things interesting and challenge your brain.

3. Mind-Body Connection: Find Your Flow

Think of these activities as a mental massage for your brain. They help you relax, de-stress, and improve your focus.

- Explore different practices: Try yoga, tai chi, meditation, or deep breathing exercises.
- Create a peaceful environment: Find a quiet space where you can focus on your practice without distractions.
- Be patient: It takes time and practice to develop mindfulness, so be kind to yourself and enjoy the journey.

4. Cognitive Training: Sharpen Your Mental Tools

Just like an athlete practices specific skills, you can train your brain with targeted activities.

- Challenge your mind: Engage in activities that require mental effort, such as learning a new language, playing brain games, or solving puzzles.
- Stay curious: Explore new hobbies, read books, or attend lectures to keep your mind active and engaged.

Make it fun: Choose activities you enjoy and that fit into your daily routine.

Remember Maria, our gardening enthusiast? Her personalized plan might include daily walks in the park, gentle yoga sessions twice a week, and challenging herself with a new Sudoku puzzle each day.

And what about our friend with early-stage Alzheimer's? He might benefit from chair exercises, water aerobics, and reminiscence therapy sessions, all tailored to his mobility level.

Fueling Your Brainpower

Don't forget to fuel your brain with a healthy diet! Think of nutritious foods as premium fuel for your brain's engine. Focus on whole grains, fruits, vegetables, lean protein, and healthy fats.

Monitoring Your Progress and Staying Motivated

Track your workouts: Use a journal, app, or fitness tracker to monitor your progress and stay accountable.
Celebrate your achievements: Acknowledge your successes and reward yourself for reaching milestones.
Find a workout buddy: Exercising with a friend or family member can provide support and motivation.
Set realistic goals: Start with small, achievable goals and gradually increase them as you get fitter.
Don't give up! There will be days when you don't feel like exercising. But remember, even a short workout is better than no workout.

The Future of Brain Training

The world of exercise and cognitive health is constantly evolving. Researchers are exploring exciting new technologies, like virtual reality exercise and personalized exercise prescriptions based on your unique needs. Stay curious and embrace the journey!

By incorporating these strategies and working closely with your healthcare team, you can harness the power of exercise to optimize your cognitive health, maintain your independence, and live a fulfilling life with diabetes. Remember, you're not just exercising your body; you're training your brain to be the best it can be!

The Brain's Sweet Tooth: Outsmarting Diabetes with a Mindful Menu

Maria stared at the swirling latte art, the foam a mocking reminder of the sugary drinks she could no longer enjoy with abandon. "Type 2 diabetes," the doctor had said, the words echoing in her mind like a death knell. It wasn't just about cutting back on sweets; it was about a future potentially clouded by cognitive decline, even dementia. Fear gnawed at her. Was this a glimpse into her golden years – a slow fade into forgetfulness?

That night, huddled under a warm blanket, Maria embarked on a frantic internet search. She found herself staring at a diagram of the brain, a complex network of pathways lit up like a city skyline. The accompanying article explained how diabetes could dim those lights, creating "traffic jams" in the brain's intricate highway system. High blood sugar, it seemed, was a recipe for cognitive disaster, starving brain cells and paving the way for conditions like Alzheimer's.

But amidst the alarming information, a glimmer of hope emerged: multimodal interventions. It wasn't just about medication; it was about a holistic approach to brain health that combined exercise, nutrition, stress management, and cognitive training. Maria, a woman who loved to dance, cook, and challenge her mind with crossword puzzles, felt a surge of empowerment. This wasn't a passive sentence; it was an invitation to take charge.

The Brain's Workout: More Than Just Flexing Muscles

Imagine your brain as a lush garden. Exercise is like the rain, nourishing the soil and helping new shoots emerge. It's not just about physical fitness; it's about boosting brainpower. Studies show that exercise:

Fine-tunes insulin sensitivity: Think of insulin as a key that unlocks the door for sugar to enter cells. Exercise helps that key work more smoothly, keeping blood sugar levels in check and preventing those brain-damaging "traffic jams."
Pumps up the cardiovascular system: Like a gardener clearing debris from a water channel, exercise strengthens the heart and improves blood flow, ensuring a steady supply of oxygen and nutrients to the brain.
Cools down inflammation: Chronic inflammation is like a wildfire in the brain, slowly damaging delicate tissues. Exercise acts like a fire extinguisher, calming the flames and protecting precious neurons.
Sprouts new brain cells: Yes, you read that right! Exercise, particularly aerobic activities like dancing or brisk walking, can stimulate the growth of new brain cells in the hippocampus, a region vital for memory and learning.
Nurtures brain-boosting chemicals: Exercise triggers the release of BDNF, a protein that acts like fertilizer for the brain, encouraging the growth and survival of neurons.

Beyond the Gym: A Mindful Menu for Brain Health

Maria signed up for a Zumba class, the vibrant music and energetic moves a welcome change from her usual sedentary routine. But she knew that exercise was just one ingredient in the recipe for a healthy brain. She started experimenting with the MIND diet, a brain-boosting blend of the Mediterranean and DASH diets, swapping sugary snacks for colorful salads and antioxidant-rich berries.

Stress Less, Remember More

Stress, Maria learned, was like a weed in her brain garden, choking the life out of her cognitive blossoms. She began incorporating mindfulness meditation into her daily routine, finding moments of stillness amidst the chaos of everyday life. The combination of exercise and stress management felt like a powerful one-two punch, clearing her mind and sharpening her focus.

Brain Games and Social Connections

Maria dusted off her old crossword puzzle books and rediscovered the joy of learning a new language. She joined a book club, finding that engaging in stimulating conversations with others was not only enjoyable but also beneficial for her cognitive health. The combination of exercise, a healthy diet, stress management, and cognitive stimulation was like a symphony for her brain, each element playing a crucial role in creating a harmonious whole.

The Future is Bright

Months later, Maria felt like a new woman. Her energy levels were up, her blood sugar was under control, and her mind felt sharper than ever. She still enjoyed the occasional sweet treat, but now it was a conscious choice, a mindful indulgence rather than a mindless habit. She knew that the journey to brain health was an ongoing one, but she faced it with confidence, armed with the knowledge and tools to protect her most precious asset – her mind.

This is just the beginning of Maria's story. What steps will you take to nourish your brain and outsmart diabetes?

Chronobiology of Exercise: Optimizing Timing for Glucose Control

The Body's Clock and Your Sugar: A Tale of Two Rhythms

Imagine your body as a bustling city, with its own intricate schedule. Delivery trucks bring supplies, construction workers repair roads, and streetlights flicker on and off, all in a carefully orchestrated rhythm. This is your circadian rhythm, your body's internal clock, and it plays a vital role in how your body handles sugar, or glucose.

The Conductor of the Orchestra: Your Circadian Rhythm

Deep in your brain, nestled in a tiny region called the suprachiasmatic nucleus (SCN), resides the master conductor of this intricate orchestra. The SCN, like a vigilant maestro, receives light signals from your eyes and synchronizes the body's internal clocks in various organs and tissues. These peripheral clocks, like skilled musicians, follow the SCN's lead but also possess their own unique rhythmicity.

At the molecular level, the circadian clock is driven by a network of core clock genes, the sheet music that guides the rhythmic expression of numerous genes involved in various physiological processes, including how your body processes sugar.

The Sugar Dance: Circadian Rhythms and Glucose Metabolism

The core clock genes, like CLOCK, BMAL1, PER, and CRY, form a complex feedback loop, a continuous dance that drives the 24-hour oscillations in gene expression. These clock genes regulate the expression of key genes involved in glucose metabolism, including those involved in insulin secretion, glucose uptake, and hepatic glucose production.

Think of BMAL1, a core clock gene, as a skilled choreographer, guiding the movements of the glucose transporter GLUT4, a crucial player in glucose uptake by muscle and adipose tissue.

Insulin's Rhythm: A Sensitive Dance Partner

Insulin sensitivity, the ability of cells to respond to insulin and take up glucose from the bloodstream, also has its own rhythm, like a dance partner attuned to the music. Insulin sensitivity is typically highest in the morning and gradually declines throughout the day, reaching its lowest point at night. This rhythm is tightly linked to the circadian clock, and disruptions to the clock can lead to missteps, impairing insulin sensitivity and contributing to insulin resistance.

When the Music Stops: Disruptions to Circadian Rhythms and Metabolic Disorders

Modern lifestyles, with their irregular sleep patterns, shift work, and exposure to artificial light at night, can disrupt the delicate balance of the circadian rhythm, like a sudden change in tempo or a missed beat. These disruptions can have profound effects on glucose metabolism and contribute to the development of metabolic disorders, including insulin resistance, metabolic syndrome, and type 2 diabetes.

Shift work, like a sudden change in time zones, disrupts the natural alignment of the circadian rhythm with the external environment. Studies have consistently shown that shift workers have an increased risk of developing metabolic disorders, including obesity, type 2 diabetes, and cardiovascular disease. The disruption of the circadian rhythm in shift workers leads to impaired glucose tolerance, decreased insulin sensitivity, and altered hormone levels, all of which contribute to metabolic dysfunction.

Sleep deprivation, another common disruptor of circadian rhythms, is like a skipped rehearsal, throwing off the timing and coordination of the body's metabolic processes. Studies have shown that even a single night of sleep deprivation can impair insulin sensitivity and glucose tolerance. Chronic sleep deprivation can lead to more severe metabolic consequences, including an increased risk of developing type 2 diabetes.

Melatonin: The Sandman's Secret Weapon

Melatonin, a hormone produced by the pineal gland in the brain, is like the sandman, promoting sleep and regulating circadian rhythms. Recent research suggests that melatonin may also have direct effects on glucose metabolism, like a secret ingredient that enhances the body's ability to handle sugar. Studies have shown that melatonin can improve insulin sensitivity and glucose tolerance, and may even protect against the development of type 2 diabetes.

Chronotherapy: Aligning Treatment with the Body's Rhythm

Chronotherapy, a therapeutic approach that takes into account the body's natural rhythms, is like adjusting the tempo and choreography to match the dancers' strengths and weaknesses. By aligning treatment schedules with the circadian rhythm, chronotherapy aims to optimize drug efficacy and minimize side effects. For example, administering insulin or other diabetes medications at specific times of the day, in sync with the body's natural insulin sensitivity rhythm, may improve glycemic control and reduce the risk of complications.

Case Studies: Real-Life Rhythms

A 45-year-old male night shift worker, whose family history was like a discordant melody, developed impaired glucose tolerance and insulin resistance. Lifestyle modifications, including regular sleep schedules, a healthy diet, and exercise, along with chronotherapy-based medication timing, helped restore harmony to his metabolic health.

A 30-year-old female with a history of sleep deprivation and irregular eating habits, like a dancer with erratic movements, developed prediabetes. Implementing a consistent sleep schedule, regular meal times, and stress management techniques led to improved glucose tolerance and prevented the progression to diabetes.

Conclusion: Keeping the Rhythm Alive

The intricate relationship between circadian rhythms and glucose metabolism highlights the importance of maintaining a healthy lifestyle that supports the body's natural rhythms. Regular sleep patterns, consistent meal times, and exposure to natural light during the day can help synchronize the circadian clock and promote metabolic health. Chronotherapy, which aligns treatment with the body's internal clock, offers a promising approach for managing metabolic disorders and optimizing patient outcomes. As research continues to unravel the complexities of this interplay, we can expect to see even more targeted and effective strategies for preventing and treating metabolic diseases.

Future Directions: The Next Movement

Personalized Chronotherapy: Developing personalized chronotherapy approaches based on individual circadian rhythms and genetic profiles, like tailoring the choreography to each dancer's unique abilities.

Novel Drug Targets: Identifying new drug targets within the molecular clock machinery to treat metabolic disorders, like discovering new instruments to enhance the orchestra's performance.

Lifestyle Interventions: Developing and implementing effective lifestyle interventions to promote circadian health and prevent metabolic dysfunction, like providing dancers with the tools and training they need to maintain their rhythm and grace.

The understanding of the interplay between circadian rhythms and glucose metabolism is rapidly evolving, opening up new avenues for research and therapeutic interventions. By harnessing the power of chronobiology, we can strive to improve metabolic health and prevent the development of diabetes and other metabolic disorders, ensuring that the body's orchestra continues to play in harmony.

Timing Your Workout for Sweet Success: A Guide to Pre-Meal Exercise for Diabetes

Imagine this: You're about to enjoy a delicious meal, but instead of feeling anxious about your blood sugar spiking, you're confident and in control. That's the power of pre-prandial exercise – a simple yet effective strategy that can transform how you manage diabetes.

Why Pre-Meal Workouts are a Game-Changer

Think of your muscles as hungry sponges, eager to soak up glucose. When you exercise before eating, you prime those sponges, making them more receptive to the glucose from your meal. This means less sugar circulating in your bloodstream, leading to:

   Tamed Blood Sugar: Say goodbye to those post-meal spikes that can leave you feeling sluggish and contribute to long-term complications.
   Boosted Insulin Power: Exercise helps your body use insulin more effectively, like giving your cells a key to unlock and absorb glucose.
   Sustained Energy: Instead of a quick burst followed by a crash, you'll enjoy steady energy levels throughout the day.

The Science Behind the Magic

Here's a peek under the hood:

   Muscle Power: When you move your body, your muscles activate special glucose transporters (imagine them as tiny doorways) that allow sugar to enter and fuel your cells.
   Insulin Efficiency: Exercise gives your insulin a helping hand, making it work smarter, not harder, to clear glucose from your blood.
   Liver Lockdown: Your liver loves to release glucose into your bloodstream, especially after meals. Pre-meal exercise helps keep your liver in check, preventing excess sugar from entering the picture.

Putting it into Practice

Ready to give pre-prandial exercise a try? Here are some tips to get you started:

Find Your Sweet Spot: Aim for moderate-intensity exercise like brisk walking, cycling, or dancing for 10-15 minutes before meals.
Listen to Your Body: If you're new to exercise or have any health concerns, talk to your doctor before starting a new routine.
Monitor Your Levels: Keep a close eye on your blood sugar before, during, and after exercise, especially when adjusting medications or trying new activities.
Make it a Habit: Consistency is key! Aim for pre-meal workouts most days of the week to reap the long-term benefits.

Beyond the Numbers

Pre-prandial exercise isn't just about managing numbers; it's about empowering you to take control of your health. It's about feeling your best, enjoying your meals without worry, and living a vibrant life with diabetes.

The Future is Personalized

As technology advances, we can expect even more personalized guidance on pre-meal exercise, tailored to your specific needs and preferences. Imagine wearable sensors that track your glucose levels and suggest the perfect workout to optimize your health.

Join the Pre-Meal Movement

Pre-prandial exercise is a simple yet powerful tool that can revolutionize your diabetes management. By incorporating it into your routine, you're not just lowering your blood sugar; you're investing in a healthier, happier future. So lace up those shoes, get moving, and experience the sweet rewards of pre-meal exercise!

Ditch the Slump: Why Your After-Dinner Stroll is a Game-Changer

We all know that exercise is good for us, but did you know that when you exercise can make a big difference? Forget the old "fasted cardio" trend – it's time to embrace the power of the post-meal power walk!

Think of it this way: you eat a meal, your blood sugar spikes, and your body scrambles to deal with it. Now imagine giving your metabolism a helping hand by getting your body moving. That's where post-prandial exercise comes in.

Why After-Dinner Exercise is Your Secret Weapon:

Sugar Superhero: When you exercise after eating, your muscles become glucose-guzzling machines, soaking up that excess sugar like a sponge. This helps prevent those nasty blood sugar spikes that can leave you feeling sluggish and wreak havoc on your health in the long run.

Insulin's Best Friend: Exercise makes your body more sensitive to insulin, the hormone that helps your cells use glucose for energy. Timing your workout for after meals gives insulin an even bigger boost, making it work smarter, not harder.

Fat-Burning Furnace: By using up readily available glucose, your body turns to its fat stores for extra fuel. This means you're not only managing your blood sugar but also torching calories and sculpting a leaner physique.

Science Says It Works!

Don't just take our word for it. Studies have shown that a simple post-meal stroll can significantly lower blood sugar levels, improve insulin sensitivity, and even help you lose weight. It's like a magic trick for your metabolism!

Ready to Get Moving? Here's the Plan:

   Timing is Everything: Aim for a 15-20 minute walk after each main meal.
   Keep it Breezy: No need to sprint! A moderate pace where you can still hold a conversation is perfect.
   Mix It Up: Walking is great, but don't be afraid to try other activities like cycling, swimming, or even dancing!
   Listen to Your Body: If you're feeling unwell or overly exhausted, skip the workout and rest.

Beyond the Basics:

The exciting thing is that scientists are still uncovering all the amazing benefits of post-meal exercise. They're exploring how different types of exercise, like strength training or HIIT, affect our metabolism after eating. Plus, with cool new tech like fitness trackers and continuous glucose monitors, we can personalize our workouts and see the results in real-time!

The Bottom Line:

Taking a walk after you eat is a simple, free, and incredibly effective way to boost your health. So ditch the after-dinner slump and embrace the power of the post-meal power walk! Your body will thank you.

   Unlock Your Fitness Superpowers: A Personalized Guide to Exercise Timing with Diabetes

Forget rigid rules and cookie-cutter plans! If you have diabetes, you know your body is unique, and your exercise routine should be too. Think of this as your personalized guide to unlocking your fitness superpowers, where you'll discover how to time your workouts for maximum energy, stable blood sugar, and a life filled with vitality.

Why Timing Matters: It's Like a Dance, Not a Battle

Imagine your body as a dance floor, with glucose as the star performer. Exercise is like the music, and insulin is the skilled choreographer. When everything's in sync, the dance is smooth and graceful. But if the music starts too early, the choreography is off, or the dancer isn't properly fueled, things can get chaotic!

That's where personalized exercise timing comes in. It's about finding the perfect rhythm for your body, so you can move with confidence and avoid those blood sugar dips and spikes that can leave you feeling drained.

Decoding Your Body's Rhythms:

Before we hit the dance floor, let's get to know your unique needs:

1. What's Your Diabetes Style?

   Type 1: The Insulin Maestro: You're the conductor of your blood sugar orchestra, relying on insulin injections to keep things in harmony. Exercise can make your cells more responsive to insulin (like giving your musicians a boost!), but it's crucial to adjust your insulin and fuel accordingly to prevent "hypo-harmonies" (aka, low blood sugar).
   Type 2: The Glucose Whisperer: You're working on improving your body's natural ability to manage glucose.

Exercise is your secret weapon, helping your cells become more efficient at using insulin and keeping blood sugar steady. But timing still matters, especially with certain medications.

2. Medication: Your Partner in the Dance

   Insulin: The Choreographer: Different types of insulin work at different speeds, so your exercise timing needs to be choreographed accordingly. Think of rapid-acting insulin as a quick-step, while long-acting insulin is more like a waltz.
   Oral Meds: The Rhythm Section: Some oral medications can make you more prone to low blood sugar during exercise, so it's important to know how they interact with your moves.

3. Fueling the Dance: What's on the Menu?

   Carbs: The Energy Boost: Carbs are like the fuel for your dance. High-glycemic carbs give you a quick burst of energy, while low-glycemic carbs provide a slower, more sustained burn.
   Protein and Fat: The Supporting Cast: These nutrients help slow down the release of glucose, preventing those sudden energy crashes.

4. Life's Rhythm: Finding Your Groove

   Work, Sleep, and Play: Your daily schedule influences when you can realistically fit in exercise. The key is to find a rhythm that works for you and your lifestyle.
   Stress: The Unwanted Guest: Stress can throw off your blood sugar and make it harder to manage during exercise. So, if you're feeling overwhelmed, opt for a relaxing activity instead of an intense workout.

Ready to Dance? Let's Create Your Personalized Routine!

(Interactive Quiz: "What's Your Exercise Timing Style?")

This quiz will ask questions about your diabetes type, medication, typical meal times, and daily schedule to help you identify your ideal exercise timing windows.

Exercise Timing Tips to Get You Moving:

Morning Movers: If you're a morning person, exercise can set the stage for stable blood sugar all day long. But be sure to check your blood sugar before and after, and adjust your insulin or fuel as needed.

Afternoon Energizers: Feeling that afternoon slump? A post-lunch workout can help regulate your blood sugar and give you a much-needed energy boost.

Evening Exercisers: Working out in the evening can be a great way to de-stress and improve your sleep. Just be mindful of how your medication and dinner affect your blood sugar overnight.

Real-Life Rhythms: Stories from the Dance Floor

Meet Maria, the Type 1 Salsa Dancer: Maria loves to dance, but her blood sugar used to dip dangerously low during her salsa classes. With the help of her doctor, she learned to adjust her insulin and fuel her body properly, and now she's dancing the night away with confidence.

Introducing Ben, the Type 2 Power Walker: Ben struggled with high blood sugar after meals until he discovered the power of a brisk walk. Now, his post-meal walks are a non-negotiable part of his routine, helping him manage his blood sugar and shed those extra pounds.

(Infographic: "Factors that Influence Your Exercise Timing")

This visually appealing infographic summarizes the key factors discussed earlier, making it easy to understand and remember.

The Future of Exercise Timing: High-Tech Harmony

Imagine a world where technology helps you fine-tune your exercise timing in real-time. With advancements like continuous glucose monitors (CGMs), AI-powered apps, and wearable sensors, this vision is becoming a reality. These tools can provide personalized insights and recommendations, making it easier than ever to find your perfect rhythm.

Embrace the Dance:

Managing diabetes can feel like a constant juggling act, but with personalized exercise timing, you can take control and find your flow. Listen to your body, experiment with different strategies, and don't be afraid to seek guidance from your healthcare team. Remember, you're not alone on this dance floor. There's a whole community of people with diabetes ready to support you every step of the way. So, put on your dancing shoes, crank up the music, and let's move!

Exercise as an Adjunct to Diabetes Technology: A Digital Revolution in Self-Management

The Future is Now: How Wearable Tech is Revolutionizing Diabetes Management

Imagine a world where managing diabetes is as easy as checking your watch. No more finger pricks, no more guessing games about your blood sugar. That's the promise of wearable sensors, and it's quickly becoming a reality.

Tiny Tech, Big Impact

These aren't your grandpa's wristwatches. We're talking about cutting-edge devices packed with sensors that track everything from your heart rate to your glucose levels in real-time. Think of it like having a mini-doctor strapped to your wrist, 24/7.

Here's how these high-tech helpers are changing the game for people with diabetes:

   Activity Tracking: Whether you're hitting the gym or just going for a walk, these devices track your every move, helping you stay active and reach your fitness goals.
   Continuous Glucose Monitoring (CGM): Say goodbye to finger pricks! CGMs continuously monitor your glucose levels, giving you a clear picture of how your body is responding to food, exercise, and medication.
   Personalized Insights: By combining data from multiple sensors, these devices provide personalized insights into your health, helping you make informed decisions about your diabetes management.

But wait, there's more!

The future of wearable tech in diabetes management is even brighter. Imagine:

AI-powered predictions: Devices that can predict high or low blood sugar events before they happen, giving you time to take action.

Closed-loop systems: A true "artificial pancreas" that automatically adjusts insulin delivery based on your glucose levels, taking the guesswork out of diabetes management.

Non-invasive glucose monitoring: No more needles! Researchers are working on devices that can measure glucose levels through the skin using light or other non-invasive methods.

The bottom line?

Wearable sensors are empowering people with diabetes to take control of their health like never before. With real-time data, personalized insights, and the potential for even more advanced features in the future, these devices are paving the way for a healthier, happier future for millions.

Imagine a world where your diabetes management isn't just about numbers on a meter, but a vibrant tapestry of data woven into the fabric of your active life. That's the power of Continuous Glucose Monitoring (CGM) – it's like having a personal glucose whisperer, guiding you towards exercise that's not just safe, but truly optimized for your body's unique rhythm.

Unleashing Your Inner Exercise Guru with CGM

Gone are the days of generic exercise advice. CGM transforms you into an exercise detective, uncovering the secrets of your glucose responses to different activities. Think of it as a personalized treasure map, revealing the sweet spot where your blood sugar dances in harmony with your workout.

Become a Glucose Detective: CGM is your magnifying glass, revealing the hidden patterns in your glucose reactions to exercise. Do you experience a steady dip during a jog, or a surprising surge during weightlifting? Armed with this knowledge, you can tailor your workouts like a bespoke suit, perfectly fitted to your individual needs.

The Workout Choreographer: CGM empowers you to curate a workout playlist that complements your glucose trends. If your levels are stable, it's time to hit the dance floor with a high-energy Zumba session. If a dip is on the horizon, a calming yoga flow might be the perfect antidote.

Timing is Everything: CGM helps you find the ideal time to exercise, like catching a wave at its peak. Exercising when your glucose is already low is like surfing a receding tide – risky and counterproductive. CGM shows you when to ride the wave of stable glucose for a smooth and exhilarating workout.

The Glucose-Balancing Act: CGM allows you to fine-tune your insulin and carb intake like a seasoned chef adjusting a delicate recipe. No more guesswork – you'll know exactly how much fuel your body needs to power through your workout and recover like a champion.

Turning Challenges into Triumphs: CGM as Your Exercise Guardian Angel

CGM isn't just about optimization; it's about safety and peace of mind. It's your vigilant guardian angel, watching over your glucose levels as you push your physical limits.

Hypoglycemia? Not on My Watch! CGM acts as your early warning system, alerting you to potential low blood sugar moments before they strike. Think of it as your glucose lifeguard, always ready to throw you a lifeline of carbs or suggest a break when needed.

Taming the Hyperglycemia Beast: If high blood sugar is your nemesis, CGM helps you harness the power of exercise to bring it back in line. It's like having a glucose-taming workout buddy, guiding you towards the right intensity and duration to achieve optimal control.

The Future is Now: Predictive Algorithms and Closed-Loop Systems

Imagine a world where your CGM not only monitors your glucose but predicts its future moves. That's the promise of cutting-edge algorithms, which analyze your past data and current trends to anticipate potential glucose swings during exercise. It's like having a glucose fortune teller, whispering secrets of your future workouts so you can stay one step ahead.

And the ultimate dream? Closed-loop systems, where your CGM and insulin pump join forces to create an automated glucose control dream team. This technology is still evolving, but it holds the potential to revolutionize exercise for people with diabetes, making glucose management as seamless as a heartbeat.

CGM: Your Passport to Exercise Freedom

CGM isn't just a tool; it's a philosophy. It's about embracing exercise, not fearing it. It's about understanding your body's unique language and using that knowledge to unlock your full athletic potential.

With CGM as your guide, you can:

Exercise with Confidence: Say goodbye to the anxiety of glucose uncertainty. CGM empowers you to push your limits, knowing you have a safety net in place.

Transform Your Relationship with Exercise: CGM reframes exercise from a chore to a celebration of your body's resilience. It's about feeling the joy of movement, not the dread of glucose complications.

Live a Fuller, More Active Life: CGM opens the door to a world of physical possibilities. Whether it's conquering a marathon or simply enjoying a walk in the park, CGM helps you embrace an active lifestyle without compromise.

The Bottom Line: CGM is more than just a glucose monitor; it's your partner in exercise optimization, your guardian angel against glucose extremes, and your passport to a life filled with movement, freedom, and confidence. So, lace up those shoes, embrace the power of CGM, and unleash your inner exercise guru!

The Rise of the Personalized Fitness Guide: How Wearables and CGMs are Revolutionizing Exercise

Imagine a world where your workout routine isn't just a generic plan, but a dynamic, ever-evolving guide tailored precisely to your body's needs. This isn't science fiction; it's the reality that's unfolding thanks to the exciting fusion of wearable technology and Continuous Glucose Monitors (CGMs).

Decoding the Body's Language: A Symphony of Data

Wearables, like fitness trackers and smartwatches, have become our constant companions, diligently recording our every move, heartbeat, and even sleep pattern. CGMs, on the other hand, provide a continuous stream of real-time glucose data, offering a crucial window into how our bodies process energy.

The true magic happens when we weave these two data streams together. It's like having a personal trainer and a nutritionist working in perfect harmony, providing a holistic view of your physiological response to exercise.

AI: The Maestro of Personalized Fitness

Artificial intelligence (AI) and machine learning algorithms take center stage in this technological symphony. They sift through mountains of data, identifying hidden patterns and correlations between your physiological parameters and glucose responses.

Think of it as having a super-smart fitness coach who can predict how your blood sugar will react to different types of exercise. This allows for the creation of bespoke workout routines that optimize your glucose control, minimizing the risk of energy crashes or spikes.

More Than Just a Workout Plan: A Dynamic Exercise Companion

But it's not just about preventing those dreaded sugar lows. AI-powered systems can craft personalized exercise plans that adapt to your fitness level, health goals, and even your glucose trends. It's like having a workout buddy who knows exactly when to push you harder and when to encourage a breather.

And if you need a little extra nudge, these systems can provide automated alerts and feedback. Imagine your smartwatch gently reminding you to grab a quick snack if your glucose levels dip during a run, or congratulating you on hitting a new personal best.

Beyond the Tech: Fostering a Love for Fitness

The integration of wearables and CGMs goes beyond just numbers and algorithms; it taps into the power of behavioral science. AI can provide personalized encouragement, making you feel like you have a cheerleader in your corner every step of the way.

Gamification adds a fun twist, turning your workouts into interactive challenges with real-time rewards. And online communities built around these technologies foster a sense of camaraderie, connecting you with like-minded individuals who share your fitness journey.

The Future of Fitness: A Glimpse into Tomorrow

While this technology is still evolving, the possibilities are endless. Imagine a future where:

- AI algorithms become so sophisticated that they can predict your body's response to exercise with incredible accuracy.
- Data integration expands to include your medical history, dietary habits, and even your stress levels, creating a truly holistic picture of your health.

Large-scale clinical trials demonstrate the undeniable benefits of this technology in improving fitness levels, blood sugar control, and overall well-being.

The Bottom Line: Your Personalized Fitness Revolution

The fusion of wearables, CGMs, and AI is ushering in a new era of personalized fitness. It's a revolution that empowers you to take control of your health, optimize your workouts, and achieve your fitness goals like never before. So, embrace the power of technology and embark on a fitness journey that's as unique as you are!

The Future of Digital Health in Diabetes Management: A Human-Centric Revolution

Imagine a world where diabetes management is seamless, intuitive, and empowering. This is the promise of digital health, a rapidly evolving field that is transforming the lives of people with diabetes. Let's explore the exciting landscape of emerging technologies and their potential to revolutionize diabetes care.

Artificial Pancreas Systems: The Intelligent Guardian

Picture a tiny device, no larger than a coin, that acts as your personal glucose guardian. This is the artificial pancreas, a closed-loop system that continuously monitors your blood sugar and automatically adjusts insulin delivery. It's like having a miniature pancreas implanted in your body, freeing you from the constant worry of managing your diabetes.

Advanced Algorithms: The Brains Behind the Operation
These systems employ sophisticated algorithms that analyze glucose trends, predict future fluctuations, and optimize insulin delivery. It's like having a personal diabetes

detective, constantly working to keep your blood sugar in check.

Integration with Continuous Glucose Monitors (CGMs): The Eyes and Ears of the System
CGMs provide real-time glucose data, allowing the artificial pancreas to make informed decisions. The latest CGMs are more accurate, comfortable, and require less frequent calibration.

Miniaturization and Wearability: Discreet and Comfortable
Researchers are working tirelessly to miniaturize the components of the artificial pancreas, making it even more discreet and comfortable to wear. Imagine a future where diabetes management is virtually invisible.

Personalized Settings: Tailored to Your Needs
Artificial pancreas systems can be customized to your individual needs and preferences, taking into account factors such as insulin sensitivity, activity levels, and meal patterns. It's like having a diabetes management system that is uniquely yours.

Clinical Trials and Implementation: Paving the Way for Wider Adoption

Promising Results: A Glimpse into the Future
Numerous clinical trials have demonstrated the efficacy and safety of artificial pancreas systems in both type 1 and type 2 diabetes. These studies have shown significant improvements in glucose control, reduced hypoglycemia, and enhanced quality of life.

Expanding Access: Breaking Down Barriers
Regulatory approvals and reimbursement policies are paving the way for wider adoption of artificial pancreas

systems. However, challenges remain in terms of cost, accessibility, and patient education.

Real-World Evidence: The Long-Term Impact
Ongoing research is gathering real-world data on the long-term effectiveness and sustainability of artificial pancreas systems in diverse populations.

Case Study: A Life Transformed

Meet Sarah, a 35-year-old woman with type 1 diabetes. Before using the artificial pancreas, she experienced frequent hypoglycemic episodes and struggled to maintain optimal glucose control. After switching to the artificial pancreas, her glucose variability significantly decreased, and she reported feeling more confident and in control of her diabetes.

Telehealth Platforms: Bridging the Gap in Diabetes Care

Imagine receiving diabetes care from the comfort of your own home. This is the power of telehealth, which utilizes various technologies, such as video conferencing, remote monitoring, and mobile apps, to connect patients with healthcare providers.

Integration with Electronic Health Records (EHRs): Seamless Data Sharing
Telehealth platforms can integrate with EHRs, allowing for seamless data sharing and care coordination. It's like having your entire diabetes care team on the same page.

Remote Patient Monitoring (RPM): Proactive Interventions
RPM devices, such as connected glucometers and blood pressure monitors, transmit data directly to healthcare providers, enabling proactive interventions

and timely adjustments to treatment plans. It's like having a virtual diabetes coach, always there to support you.

Patient-Facing Apps: Empowering Self-Management

Mobile apps provide patients with tools for self-management, including glucose tracking, medication reminders, educational resources, and communication with healthcare providers. It's like having a diabetes management toolkit at your fingertips.

Artificial Intelligence (AI)-Powered Chatbots: 24/7 Support

AI-powered chatbots can provide personalized guidance, answer questions, and offer support to patients 24/7. It's like having a diabetes expert available at any time of day or night.

Clinical Trials and Implementation: Expanding Access and Improving Outcomes

Improved Access and Outcomes: Reaching Underserved Populations

Studies have shown that telehealth interventions can improve glucose control, reduce hospitalizations, and enhance patient satisfaction.

Cost-Effectiveness: Optimizing Healthcare Resources

Telehealth can be a cost-effective way to deliver diabetes care, particularly for patients in rural areas or those with limited access to specialized care.

Integration into Healthcare Systems: The Future of Care Delivery

Healthcare systems are increasingly incorporating telehealth into their care models, recognizing its potential to improve access, quality, and efficiency of care.

Case Study: Breaking Down Geographical Barriers

Meet John, a 60-year-old man with type 2 diabetes living in a rural area. Through video consultations and remote monitoring, he received regular check-ups, medication adjustments, and lifestyle counseling from his healthcare provider. This program helped him achieve better glucose control and avoid unnecessary trips to the clinic.

Virtual Reality Exercise Programs: Making Fitness Fun and Engaging

Imagine exercising in a virtual world, surrounded by breathtaking scenery and motivational challenges. This is the promise of virtual reality (VR) technology, which is gaining traction as an innovative tool for promoting physical activity and exercise adherence in individuals with diabetes.

Interactive Environments: Immersive and Engaging

VR headsets create immersive environments that simulate real-world scenarios, such as walking through a park or cycling through a scenic route. It's like exercising in a different world.

Gamification: Making Fitness Fun

VR exercise programs often incorporate gamification elements, such as rewards, challenges, and leaderboards, to enhance motivation and engagement. It's like turning exercise into a game.

Personalized Workouts: Tailored to Your Fitness Level

VR systems can adapt workouts to individual fitness levels and preferences, providing customized exercise plans. It's like having a personal trainer in your VR headset.

Social Interaction: Exercising with Friends and Family

Some VR platforms allow users to exercise with friends or family members in virtual environments, fostering social support and motivation. It's like having a workout buddy, even if they're miles away.

Clinical Trials and Implementation: The Future of Fitness

Improved Fitness and Glycemic Control: The Benefits of VR Exercise
Preliminary studies suggest that VR exercise programs can improve cardiorespiratory fitness, increase physical activity levels, and enhance glucose control in individuals with diabetes.

Enhanced Motivation and Adherence: Making Exercise a Habit
The immersive and engaging nature of VR can motivate individuals to exercise more regularly and adhere to their fitness goals.

Accessibility and Convenience: Exercising from Anywhere
VR exercise programs can be accessed from the comfort of one's home, eliminating barriers such as transportation and weather.

Case Study: Overcoming Exercise Barriers

Meet Lisa, a 45-year-old woman with type 2 diabetes who struggled to maintain a consistent exercise routine due to lack of motivation and time constraints. She enrolled in a VR exercise program that offered interactive cycling tours through scenic landscapes. The immersive experience and gamification elements kept her engaged and motivated, leading to increased physical activity and improved glucose control.

Conclusion: A Brighter Future for Diabetes Management

The future of digital health in diabetes management is bright, with emerging technologies poised to revolutionize care and empower individuals to live healthier lives. Artificial pancreas systems, telehealth platforms, and virtual reality exercise programs offer innovative solutions for improving glucose control, promoting healthy behaviors, and enhancing quality of life. As these technologies continue to evolve and become more accessible, they hold the potential to transform the landscape of diabetes care and improve outcomes for millions of people worldwide.

Research Focus: Shaping the Future of Digital Health

Technological Advancements: Refining and Optimizing Technologies
Ongoing research is crucial to further refine and optimize these technologies, enhancing their accuracy, effectiveness, and user-friendliness.

Clinical Trials: Evaluating Long-Term Safety and Efficacy
Rigorous clinical trials are needed to evaluate the long-term safety and efficacy of these technologies in diverse populations and real-world settings.

Implementation Science: Understanding Adoption Factors
Research is needed to understand the factors that influence the successful implementation and adoption of these technologies in healthcare systems.

Health Economics: Determining Value and Affordability

Cost-effectiveness analyses are essential to determine the value and affordability of these technologies for individuals and healthcare systems.

By fostering innovation, conducting rigorous research, and promoting collaboration, we can harness the full potential of digital health to transform diabetes care and improve the lives of individuals with diabetes.

High-Intensity Interval Training (HIIT): A Time-Efficient Strategy for Diabetes Management

Unleashing the Power Within: HIIT and the Diabetic Body

Imagine a workout that not only strengthens your heart but also empowers your body to better manage diabetes. That's the magic of High-Intensity Interval Training (HIIT). Think of it as a superhero workout – short bursts of intense activity that push your limits, followed by moments of recovery, like a superhero recharging for their next battle.

Revving Up Your Inner Engine: Cardiorespiratory Fitness

HIIT is like a turbo boost for your heart and lungs. It pushes your body to use oxygen more efficiently, making your cardiovascular system a well-oiled machine. Studies show that HIIT can significantly improve cardiorespiratory fitness in people with diabetes, even more so than traditional moderate-intensity exercise. This means more energy for everyday activities and a reduced risk of heart complications.

Powering Up Your Cells: Mitochondrial Function

Mitochondria are the tiny powerhouses within our cells, responsible for producing energy. HIIT acts like a personal trainer for your mitochondria, making them more numerous and efficient. This is especially important for people with diabetes, as it helps improve how their body uses glucose and responds to insulin.

Unlocking the Glucose Gateway: Glucose Transport

Glucose is like fuel for our bodies, and HIIT helps unlock the doors to let that fuel into our cells. It increases the production of GLUT4, a protein that acts like a gatekeeper for glucose, allowing it to enter muscle cells more easily. This helps regulate blood sugar levels and prevents those dangerous spikes.

Sharpening Your Insulin Response: Insulin Sensitivity

Insulin is like a key that unlocks the door for glucose to enter cells. In diabetes, this lock can become rusty. HIIT acts like a lubricant, improving insulin sensitivity and allowing the body to use insulin more effectively. This means better blood sugar control and potentially less reliance on medication.

Real-Life Heroes: Examples and Case Studies

A recent study published in "Diabetes Care" showed that people with type 2 diabetes who did HIIT experienced a greater improvement in their fitness levels compared to those who did moderate-intensity exercise.

Imagine a 55-year-old man with type 2 diabetes who starts a HIIT program. After 12 weeks, his fitness improves dramatically, his blood sugar levels are under better control, and he even reduces his insulin dosage. This is the power of HIIT in action.

HIIT: A Powerful Ally in Diabetes Management

HIIT is more than just a workout; it's a way to empower your body to better manage diabetes. By improving cardiorespiratory fitness, boosting mitochondrial function, enhancing glucose transport, and sharpening insulin sensitivity, HIIT offers a unique and effective approach to improving health and well-being.

Important Note: Always consult your doctor before starting any new exercise program, especially if you have diabetes or any other health conditions.

HIIT vs. MICT: The Ultimate Showdown for Diabetes Management

Imagine your body as a car. Moderate-intensity continuous training (MICT) is like a leisurely drive down the highway – you're cruising along, burning fuel at a steady pace. High-intensity interval training (HIIT), on the other hand, is like a thrilling race car circuit – bursts of intense speed followed by pit stops. Both get you where you need to go, but which is the best route for managing diabetes?

That's the burning question this research review tackles! We dug deep into the science, comparing HIIT and MICT head-to-head to see which one reigns supreme in managing blood sugar, boosting heart health, and improving overall quality of life for people with type 1 and type 2 diabetes.

What We Found:

Blood Sugar Control: Both HIIT and MICT are like superheroes for your blood sugar, effectively lowering HbA1c (average blood sugar levels). But when it comes to those pesky blood sugar swings, HIIT emerges as the champion, keeping your levels steadier than a tightrope walker.

Heart Health: Both workouts are like a spa day for your heart, lowering blood pressure and improving cholesterol.

However, HIIT gives your systolic blood pressure (the top number) an extra powerful punch.

   Quality of Life: Feeling good is just as important as numbers! Both HIIT and MICT boost your physical abilities and mental well-being. But if you're looking to become a stair-climbing ninja, HIIT might be your secret weapon.

The Verdict:

It's a tie! Both HIIT and MICT are fantastic for managing diabetes. The best choice for you depends on your personal preferences, fitness level, and goals.

Think of it this way:

   Love variety and quick workouts? HIIT might be your jam.
   Prefer a steady pace and enjoy longer sessions? MICT could be your perfect match.

The Bottom Line:

Whether you choose the thrilling race car or the scenic route, the most important thing is to get moving! Talk to your doctor about which exercise plan is right for you and start experiencing the amazing benefits.

Real-Life Examples:

   The Busy Executive: John, a 50-year-old with type 2 diabetes, finds it hard to squeeze in exercise. HIIT is his solution – quick, effective workouts that fit his hectic schedule.
   The Zen Master: Maria, a 35-year-old with type 1 diabetes, prefers the calming rhythm of MICT. Her daily walks help her manage stress and keep her blood sugar in check.

The Future of Diabetes Management:

This research gives us a clearer picture of how exercise impacts diabetes, but there's still more to discover! Scientists are continuing to explore the long-term effects of HIIT and MICT, the ideal workout routines for different people, and how these exercise styles work their magic on the body.

The Takeaway:

No matter which path you choose, exercise is a powerful tool for managing diabetes and living a healthier, happier life. So, lace up those shoes and get moving!

Unleashing Your Inner Powerhouse: A HIIT Guide for Diabetes

Imagine this: You're not just managing diabetes, you're thriving with it. You're bursting with energy, your blood sugar is in check, and you feel amazing. That's the power of HIIT (High-Intensity Interval Training), a workout style that's like a secret weapon for people with diabetes.

Why HIIT is Your Diabetes Superhero

Think of HIIT as a turbo boost for your body. It's all about short bursts of intense exercise followed by quick rests. This "go hard, then chill" approach does wonders for your blood sugar, helps your body use insulin better, and even torches calories. It's like hitting the fast-forward button on your fitness goals!

HIIT and Diabetes: A Dynamic Duo

HIIT is a game-changer for diabetes, but it's important to do it right. Here's the lowdown:

Intensity is Key: Aim for a workout that feels like an 8 or 9 on a scale of 1 to 10. Think sprints, burpees, or jumping jacks – anything that gets your heart pumping!

Listen to Your Body: Start with shorter intervals (around 30 seconds) and gradually increase the time as you get fitter. Always prioritize rest and recovery.

Mix It Up: Variety is the spice of life, and HIIT is no different. Try different exercises like cycling, swimming, or even dancing to keep things interesting.

Safety First: Check with your doctor before starting any new workout routine, especially if you have any other health conditions. Keep a close eye on your blood sugar levels and stay hydrated.

HIIT in Action: Real-Life Success Stories

Mark's Transformation: Mark, a 55-year-old with type 2 diabetes, was tired of feeling sluggish. He started a HIIT program with cycling intervals and saw his blood sugar, blood pressure, and fitness levels improve dramatically.

Sarah's Journey: Sarah, a 40-year-old with type 1 diabetes, found that HIIT helped her manage her blood sugar and even reduced nerve pain. She started with modified bodyweight exercises and gradually increased the intensity as she got stronger.

The Bottom Line

HIIT is a powerful tool for people with diabetes, but it's important to approach it with a personalized plan. Listen to your body, work with your doctor, and get ready to unlock a healthier, more energetic you.

Subtopic 4: Integrating HIIT into Clinical Practice: A Practical Guide for Healthcare Professionals

This section provides comprehensive guidance for healthcare professionals on incorporating High-Intensity Interval Training (HIIT) into diabetes management plans. It covers patient assessment, exercise counseling, progression strategies, and addressing potential barriers to adherence, with a focus on behavioral interventions, motivational strategies, and clinical implementation.

Patient Assessment

Before recommending HIIT, a thorough patient assessment is crucial to ensure safety and effectiveness. This assessment should include:

Medical History:

Diabetes Type and Control: Assess the type of diabetes (Type 1, Type 2, or other), disease duration, current blood glucose control (HbA1c levels), and history of hypoglycemia or hyperglycemia.
Cardiovascular Health: Evaluate cardiovascular risk factors such as blood pressure, cholesterol levels, and any history of heart disease, stroke, or peripheral artery disease.
Other Medical Conditions: Identify any other health conditions that may affect exercise participation, such as arthritis, kidney disease, or neuropathy.
Medications: Review the patient's medication list, including insulin or other diabetes medications, as these can influence exercise responses and blood glucose levels.

Physical Fitness:

Cardiorespiratory Fitness: Assess aerobic capacity using a graded exercise test or submaximal test if available. Consider alternative assessments like the 6-minute walk test for patients with limitations.
Musculoskeletal Fitness: Evaluate muscle strength and endurance, flexibility, and balance. Identify any physical limitations or pain that may affect exercise performance.
Body Composition: Measure body mass index (BMI) and waist circumference to assess obesity-related risks.

Lifestyle and Preferences:

Physical Activity Level: Determine the patient's current physical activity habits and exercise experience.
Lifestyle Factors: Assess dietary habits, sleep patterns, stress levels, and social support, as these can influence exercise adherence.
Preferences and Goals: Discuss the patient's exercise preferences, goals, and any concerns or barriers they anticipate.

Example Case:

A 55-year-old male with Type 2 diabetes for 10 years presents with an HbA1c of 8.5%. He has hypertension, dyslipidemia, and a sedentary lifestyle. Physical assessment reveals obesity (BMI 32 kg/m²), decreased aerobic capacity, and limited flexibility. He expresses interest in trying HIIT but is concerned about his knee pain and lack of time.

Exercise Counseling

After the assessment, provide personalized exercise counseling to educate the patient about HIIT and develop a safe and effective exercise plan.

Explain HIIT:

Concept: Describe HIIT as involving short bursts of high-intensity exercise followed by brief recovery periods.
Benefits: Emphasize the benefits of HIIT for diabetes management, including improved blood glucose control, cardiovascular health, and weight management.
Safety: Address any concerns about safety, emphasizing the importance of proper warm-up, cool-down, and individualized exercise intensity.

Develop an Individualized Plan:

Exercise Prescription: Based on the assessment, prescribe a HIIT program with appropriate exercise modalities, intensity, duration, and frequency. Consider starting with low-impact activities and gradually increasing intensity and duration.
Blood Glucose Monitoring: Advise the patient on blood glucose monitoring before, during, and after exercise, especially when starting a new program or adjusting medications.
Hydration and Nutrition: Emphasize the importance of adequate hydration and proper nutrition to support exercise performance and blood glucose control.

Address Potential Barriers:

Time Constraints: Explore strategies for incorporating HIIT into a busy schedule, such as shorter workouts or utilizing available resources like online videos or community programs.

Physical Limitations: Modify exercises to accommodate physical limitations or pain. Consider alternative activities like water-based exercises or chair-based exercises.

Lack of Motivation: Discuss motivational strategies, such as setting realistic goals, finding an exercise buddy, or using technology to track progress and provide feedback.

Example Case (Continued):

The patient is educated about HIIT and its benefits for diabetes management. His exercise plan starts with low-impact activities like brisk walking and cycling, gradually incorporating higher-intensity intervals. He is advised to monitor blood glucose regularly and adjust his medication as needed. Strategies for overcoming time constraints and managing knee pain are discussed, and he is encouraged to set realistic goals and track his progress.

Progression Strategies

As the patient adapts to HIIT, gradually progress the exercise program to maintain challenge and optimize benefits.

Intensity: Gradually increase the intensity of the high-intensity intervals by increasing speed, resistance, or incline. Shorten the recovery periods between intervals to increase the overall intensity. Incorporate different levels of intensity within a workout to provide variety and challenge.

Duration: Gradually increase the duration of the high-intensity intervals. Add more intervals or sets to the workout.

Frequency: Gradually increase the number of HIIT sessions per week.

Modality: Introduce new exercises to target different muscle groups and maintain interest. Progress to higher-impact activities like running or jumping if appropriate.

Example Case (Continued):

After 4 weeks of consistent HIIT, the patient's fitness improves, and his blood glucose control shows positive trends. His exercise plan is progressed by increasing the intensity and duration of intervals, incorporating new exercises like bodyweight circuits, and adding an extra HIIT session per week. He is motivated by his progress and continues to adhere to the program.

Addressing Potential Barriers to Adherence

Despite the benefits of HIIT, adherence can be challenging. Proactively address potential barriers to support long-term success.

Behavioral Interventions:

Goal Setting: Help the patient set realistic and achievable goals, breaking down larger goals into smaller, manageable steps.

Self-Monitoring: Encourage the use of logs, journals, or wearable technology to track exercise progress and identify patterns or triggers for lapses.

Problem-Solving: Collaboratively address challenges and develop solutions to overcome barriers, such as scheduling conflicts, lack of social support, or weather limitations.

Relapse Prevention: Discuss strategies for managing setbacks and preventing relapse, such as identifying high-risk situations and developing coping mechanisms.

Motivational Strategies:

Positive Reinforcement: Provide positive feedback and encouragement to reinforce progress and maintain motivation.

Social Support: Encourage the patient to find an exercise buddy or join a support group to enhance motivation and accountability.

Intrinsic Motivation: Explore activities the patient enjoys and help them connect exercise to their personal values and goals.

Mindfulness and Enjoyment: Encourage the patient to focus on the present moment and find activities they enjoy to enhance exercise adherence.

Clinical Implementation:

Interdisciplinary Approach: Collaborate with other healthcare professionals, such as dietitians, certified diabetes educators, and mental health professionals, to provide comprehensive care.

Technology Integration: Utilize telehealth, mobile apps, and wearable technology to provide remote support, monitor progress, and enhance engagement.

Community Resources: Refer patients to community-based programs, fitness centers, or online resources to support their exercise goals.

Follow-up and Support: Schedule regular follow-up appointments to monitor progress, address concerns, and adjust the exercise plan as needed.

Example Case (Continued):

The patient experiences a setback due to work travel and struggles to maintain his exercise routine. His healthcare team provides support through telehealth check-ins, helps him adjust his exercise plan, and encourages him to utilize online resources for workouts while traveling. He successfully overcomes the setback and continues to progress towards his goals.

Conclusion

Integrating HIIT into clinical practice requires a comprehensive approach that includes thorough patient assessment, individualized exercise counseling, progressive strategies, and proactive management of potential barriers. By utilizing behavioral interventions, motivational strategies, and effective clinical implementation, healthcare professionals can empower individuals with diabetes to safely and effectively incorporate HIIT into their diabetes management plans, leading to improved health outcomes and quality of life.

Exercise as a Countermeasure to Diabetic Neuropathy

Imagine a world where your body is a symphony orchestra, each organ playing its part in a harmonious concert. Now, imagine a conductor who's lost their baton, the music becoming discordant, the instruments falling out of tune. This is the unsettling reality of diabetic neuropathy, a condition where high blood sugar levels wreak havoc on the nervous system, like a relentless maestro leading the body astray.

Peripheral Neuropathy: The Silent Thief of Sensation

Imagine walking on a bed of needles, or perhaps not feeling anything at all. This is the cruel irony of peripheral neuropathy, the most common form of nerve damage in diabetes. It's like a thief in the night, slowly stealing away your sense of touch, leaving behind a trail of numbness, tingling, and burning pain. It can even rob you of your balance, making every step a gamble.

The culprit? High blood sugar, a relentless saboteur that sets off a chain reaction of damage. It's like a flood that engulfs the nerves, leaving behind a sticky residue called advanced glycation end products (AGEs). These AGEs are like tiny gremlins, causing inflammation and oxidative stress, disrupting the delicate balance of the nervous system.

Autonomic Neuropathy: The Body's Control Center Under Siege

Imagine a control center where the lights flicker, the buttons malfunction, and the signals get crossed. This is the chaotic scene in autonomic neuropathy, where the nerves that regulate our vital functions come under attack. It's like a power outage in the body, leaving us vulnerable to a host of problems.

The heart races uncontrollably, the stomach churns with nausea, and the bladder loses its grip. Even the pupils, those windows to the soul, become sluggish and unresponsive. It's a domino effect of dysfunction, as the body struggles to maintain its delicate equilibrium.

Proximal Neuropathy: The Unexpected Attack

Imagine a sudden, sharp pain that shoots through your hip and thigh, leaving you weak and unable to move. This is the unwelcome surprise of proximal neuropathy, a less common but equally debilitating form of nerve damage. It's like a lightning strike, leaving behind a trail of pain, weakness, and muscle wasting.

The exact cause remains a mystery, but high blood sugar and inflammation are likely suspects. It's a reminder that diabetes is a relentless foe, always lurking in the shadows, ready to strike when we least expect it.

The Future of Diabetic Neuropathy: A Glimmer of Hope

Despite the challenges, there's hope on the horizon. Researchers are working tirelessly to unravel the mysteries of diabetic neuropathy, searching for new treatments and cures. They're exploring innovative therapies, from nerve regeneration to gene editing, in the quest to restore balance and harmony to the body's symphony.

In the meantime, the best defense is a good offense. By managing blood sugar levels, adopting a healthy lifestyle, and seeking early intervention, we can reduce the risk of diabetic neuropathy and protect our precious nervous system. After all, a well-conducted orchestra is a joy to behold, and a healthy body is a symphony worth preserving.

The Power of Exercise: Your Body's Natural Nerve Protector

Unleashing the Healing Potential of Movement

Picture your nerves as a bustling network of wires, carrying vital messages between your brain and body. Now imagine these wires damaged, causing tingling, numbness, and pain – the hallmarks of diabetic neuropathy. But what if there was a way to repair these damaged wires, to restore the lost connection and alleviate the debilitating symptoms?

Enter the world of exercise, a natural healer with the potential to revolutionize the management of diabetic neuropathy. In this article, we'll explore how exercise works its magic, protecting your nerves from further damage and potentially even promoting regeneration.

Exercise: More Than Just a Workout

When you exercise, you're not just pumping iron or sweating it out at the gym; you're also engaging in a symphony of physiological changes that benefit your entire body, including your nervous system.

1. Boosting Blood Flow to Your Nerves

Think of your nerves like a city's electrical grid. Just as a city needs a steady supply of power to function, your nerves need a steady supply of oxygen and nutrients to thrive. Exercise helps improve blood flow to your nerves in several ways:

Widening blood vessels: Exercise relaxes the muscles surrounding your blood vessels, allowing them to dilate and increase blood flow. This is like opening up the city's streets to accommodate more traffic.

Creating new blood vessels: Regular exercise can stimulate the growth of new blood vessels in your nerves, further enhancing blood flow and nutrient delivery. This is like building new roads to reduce traffic congestion.

Improved blood flow ensures that your nerves get the nourishment they need to stay healthy and function properly.

2. Fighting Oxidative Stress

When blood sugar levels are chronically high, it can lead to a buildup of harmful molecules called reactive oxygen species (ROS). These molecules can damage nerve cells and contribute to the development of diabetic neuropathy.

Exercise acts as a powerful antioxidant, neutralizing ROS and protecting your nerves from damage. It does this by:

Increasing the production of antioxidants: Exercise stimulates the production of enzymes that scavenge ROS, like superoxide dismutase and catalase. These enzymes act like firefighters, extinguishing the ROS before they can cause damage.

Improving mitochondrial function: Mitochondria are the powerhouses of your cells, responsible for energy production. Exercise can improve mitochondrial function, reducing their production of ROS and promoting healthy energy metabolism.

By reducing oxidative stress, exercise helps to preserve the structure and function of your nerves.

3. Promoting Nerve Growth and Repair

Exercise can also stimulate the production of neurotrophic factors, proteins that promote the growth, survival, and function of nerve cells. These factors play a crucial role in nerve regeneration and repair.

Studies have shown that exercise can increase the levels of neurotrophic factors like nerve growth factor (NGF) and brain-derived neurotrophic factor (BDNF) in the blood and in nerve tissue. This can help to:

   Repair damaged nerves: NGF and BDNF can stimulate the growth of new nerve fibers and promote the repair of damaged ones.
   Protect existing nerves: These factors can also help to protect existing nerves from further damage and maintain their function.

By promoting nerve growth and repair, exercise can help to restore lost nerve function and improve symptoms of diabetic neuropathy.

Types of Exercise That Benefit Your Nerves

Most types of exercise can benefit your nerves, but some may be more effective than others. Here are a few to consider:

   Aerobic exercise: Activities like walking, jogging, cycling, and swimming are great for improving overall cardiovascular health and increasing blood flow to your nerves.

Strength training: Resistance training can help to build muscle strength and improve balance, which can indirectly benefit your nerves by reducing the risk of falls and injuries.

Balance and coordination exercises: These exercises can help to improve your balance and coordination, reducing your risk of falls and further nerve damage.

Talk to Your Doctor Before Starting Any New Exercise Program

Before starting any new exercise program, it's important to talk to your doctor. They can help you create a safe and effective exercise plan that's right for you and your individual health needs.

Exercise: Your Path to Nerve Health

If you're living with diabetes, exercise is a powerful tool that can help you protect your nerves and improve your quality of life. By incorporating regular exercise into your routine, you can take control of your health and pave the way for a brighter future.

Remember, every step you take is a step towards a healthier you!

Subtopic 3: Exercise Prescriptions for Neuropathy Management

Imagine your nerves are like tiny wires sending signals throughout your body. With diabetic neuropathy, these wires get frayed and damaged, causing pain, numbness, and balance problems. But there's good news! Exercise can act like a repair crew, helping to mend those wires and restore their function.

Exercise: Your Body's Electrician

Think of exercise as your body's electrician, rewiring and re-energizing your nervous system. It gets your blood pumping, delivering oxygen and nutrients to those damaged nerves. It strengthens your muscles, providing better support and balance. And it even encourages your body to create new nerve connections, like building new pathways for signals to travel.

The Exercise Prescription

Just like a doctor prescribes medicine, we can prescribe exercise for neuropathy. Here's what the research tells us:

   Aerobic Exercise: Get your heart pumping with brisk walking, dancing, swimming, or cycling. Aim for at least 30 minutes most days of the week.
   Strength Training: Build muscle power with weights, resistance bands, or bodyweight exercises. Focus on all major muscle groups 2-3 times a week.
   Balance Training: Improve your stability with tai chi, yoga, or simple exercises like standing on one leg. Practice a few times a week.
   Flexibility Exercises: Keep your body limber with stretching and range-of-motion exercises. Hold each stretch for 15-30 seconds and repeat several times.

Listen to Your Body

Remember, everyone's body is different. Start slowly and gradually increase the intensity and duration of your exercise. Pay attention to your body's signals and don't overdo it. If you experience pain, stop and rest.

Real-Life Success Stories

    A 60-year-old man with neuropathy joined a 12-week exercise program. He found his pain decreased, his balance improved, and he could enjoy activities he once struggled with.
    A 55-year-old woman with neuropathy started tai chi. She felt more stable, coordinated, and had a greater sense of well-being.
    A 65-year-old man with neuropathy combined aerobic and strength training. He noticed less pain, improved numbness, and better blood sugar control.

Exercise: Your Path to a Better Life

Exercise is not just about managing symptoms; it's about improving your overall quality of life. It can boost your mood, reduce stress, and help you sleep better. It can empower you to take control of your health and live a more fulfilling life.

Important Note: Always consult your doctor before starting any new exercise program, especially if you have diabetic neuropathy. They can help you create a personalized plan that's safe and effective for you.

Remember: You are not alone. With the right exercise plan and support, you can manage your neuropathy and live a vibrant, active life.

Would you like to explore specific exercises or learn more about managing diabetic neuropathy?

Neuropathy: When Your Body Betrays You (But You Can Fight Back!)

Imagine waking up every morning with your feet feeling like they're wrapped in burning coals, or trying to button your shirt with fingers that feel like they're wearing thick gloves even on a summer day. This is the reality for many people with diabetic neuropathy, a common complication of diabetes that turns your own nerves against you.

But don't despair! While neuropathy can be a formidable foe, it's not invincible. By understanding this condition and embracing a holistic approach to care, you can reclaim your life and live vibrantly, even with neuropathy. Deciphering the Enemy: What is Diabetic Neuropathy?

Think of your nerves as a vast communication network, constantly sending signals throughout your body. Diabetes, with its relentless high blood sugar, acts like a saboteur, damaging these vital pathways. This can lead to a range of symptoms that vary depending on which nerves are affected:

   Sensory Neuropathy: The Phantom Menace: This is where the "burning feet" sensation comes into play, along with numbness, tingling, or shooting pains in your hands and feet. Imagine trying to walk on hot sand or pick up a delicate object with numb fingers – everyday tasks become a minefield of discomfort.
   Motor Neuropathy: The Puppet Master: This form of neuropathy weakens your muscles, making it difficult to move with ease and coordination. Simple actions like climbing stairs or even walking can become herculean efforts, increasing your risk of falls and injuries.
   Autonomic Neuropathy: The Silent Saboteur: This sneaky form of neuropathy disrupts the automatic functions of

your body, like digestion, heart rate, blood pressure, and sweating. It's like having a gremlin messing with your internal control panel, leading to problems like dizziness, digestive issues, and even heart complications.

Exercise: Your Secret Weapon Against Neuropathy

Now, for the good news! Exercise isn't just about getting fit; it's a powerful weapon in your arsenal against neuropathy. Think of it as your body's own repair crew, working tirelessly to restore those damaged communication lines and reclaim your well-being. Here's how:

    Taming the Sugar Beast: When you move your body, you're giving your insulin a helping hand. It's like turning up the volume on a radio signal, allowing your cells to hear the message loud and clear and use that energy effectively. This helps keep your blood sugar in check and protects your nerves from further damage. (Image of a person enjoying a brisk walk outdoors)
    Rewiring the Network: Remember those frayed telephone wires? Exercise helps repair them! It promotes nerve regeneration and improves nerve conduction velocity, which is like boosting the signal strength and clarity. This can lead to a reduction in those pesky symptoms like numbness and tingling.
    Fueling the Front Lines: Exercise gets your blood pumping, delivering essential nutrients and oxygen to those damaged nerves. It's like sending in a supply convoy to support the repair efforts and soothe the inflammation causing your pain.
    The Endorphin Rush: Ever felt that "runner's high"? That's the power of endorphins, your body's natural painkillers. Exercise triggers their release, providing much-needed relief from neuropathic pain.
    Finding Your Balance: Specific exercises can help you regain your balance and coordination, like a tightrope

walker finding their footing. This reduces your risk of falls and helps you move with confidence.

The Whole-Body Boost: Exercise doesn't just benefit your nerves; it improves your overall health. It strengthens your heart, helps you manage your weight, and even lifts your mood. It's like giving your entire body a tune-up!

Meet Maria: Maria, a vibrant 62-year-old with type 2 diabetes, was devastated when neuropathy started robbing her of her independence. Simple tasks like walking her dog or gardening became agonizing. But Maria refused to be defeated. She started with gentle exercises like chair yoga and short walks, gradually increasing her activity level as her symptoms improved. Today, Maria is back to tending her beloved garden and enjoying long walks with her furry companion. Exercise gave her back her freedom.

Exercise for Psychological Well-being in Diabetes

The Mind-Body Tango: When Diabetes and Mental Health Collide

Imagine your body and mind as dance partners. Ideally, they move together with grace and ease. But sometimes, they step on each other's toes, leading to a clumsy and frustrating dance. That's what happens when diabetes and mental health conditions like depression and anxiety get tangled up.

The Vicious Cycle

Think of it like a seesaw. When diabetes acts up, it can weigh down your mental health, making you feel stressed, anxious, or even depressed. On the flip side, if you're struggling with your mental health, it can throw your diabetes management off balance, leading to higher blood sugar levels and a greater risk of complications.

Diabetes Distress: The Emotional Baggage of Diabetes

Living with diabetes can be like carrying around a heavy suitcase filled with worries, frustrations, and "what ifs." This emotional burden is called diabetes distress, and it can make it even harder to keep up with the demands of managing your condition.

The Case of the Vanishing Motivation

Imagine you're trying to climb a mountain, but the weight of diabetes distress is pulling you down. You feel exhausted, overwhelmed, and like giving up. This can lead to neglecting your diabetes care, like skipping medication or making unhealthy food choices.

The Fear Factor

Anxiety can be a sneaky saboteur when it comes to diabetes management. It can whisper doubts in your ear, making you afraid of needles, blood sugar checks, or even the possibility of complications. This fear can paralyze you, making it hard to take the necessary steps to stay healthy.

Breaking the Cycle, Finding the Rhythm

The good news is that you can learn to dance with diabetes and mental health challenges in a way that feels more harmonious. Here are a few steps to help you find your rhythm:

   Talk It Out: Don't suffer in silence. Share your struggles with your doctor, a therapist, or a support group. Talking about your feelings can help you feel less alone and find healthy ways to cope.

   Mindful Moments: Take a break from the diabetes dance floor and practice mindfulness. Meditation, deep breathing, or simply spending time in nature can help you calm your mind and reconnect with your body.

   Teamwork Makes the Dream Work: Build a support team of healthcare providers, family, and friends who can cheer you on and offer a helping hand when you need it.

   Celebrate Small Victories: Focus on the progress you're making, no matter how small. Each step you take towards better diabetes and mental health management is a reason to celebrate.

Remember, you're not alone in this dance. With the right support and a little self-compassion, you can find your rhythm and move towards a healthier, happier you.

Exercise: Your Mental Health's Secret Weapon

Ever feel down or anxious? Exercise might be the answer you're looking for. It's not just for your body; it's a powerful tool for boosting your mental well-being.

The Science Behind Exercise and Mental Health

When you exercise, your brain releases chemicals called endorphins, often referred to as the "feel-good" hormones. These endorphins interact with receptors in your brain to reduce feelings of pain and improve mood.

But that's not all. Exercise also plays a role in regulating other important neurotransmitters like serotonin, dopamine, and norepinephrine, which are involved in mood, sleep, and stress response.

How Exercise Can Help with Depression and Anxiety

Studies have shown that regular exercise can significantly reduce symptoms of depression and anxiety. In fact, it can be as effective as medication or therapy in some cases.

One study found that people with depression who exercised for just 30 minutes three times a week experienced a significant improvement in their symptoms after six weeks. Another study found that exercise was as effective as antidepressants in reducing anxiety symptoms in people with generalized anxiety disorder.

Beyond Mood Boosting: Exercise and Neuroplasticity

Exercise not only improves your mood but also has a positive impact on your brain structure and function. It can increase the growth of new brain cells, strengthen existing connections between neurons, and improve blood flow to the brain.

These changes can lead to improved cognitive function, memory, and learning.

Getting Started

If you're looking to improve your mental health through exercise, there are a few things to keep in mind:

   Start slow and gradually increase the intensity and duration of your workouts.
   Choose activities you enjoy.
   Find a workout buddy or join a fitness class for extra motivation.

It's also important to be patient. It may take a few weeks or even months to see a significant improvement in your mental health. But with consistent effort, you'll be well on your way to a happier, healthier you.

Remember, exercise is not only good for your body; it's also good for your mind. So lace up your sneakers and get moving!

   Imagine this:

You're sitting across from a friend, a warm cup of tea in your hands. They've recently been diagnosed with diabetes and feel overwhelmed. Not just by the physical challenges, but by a creeping sense of anxiety and low mood they just can't shake. You listen with empathy, then share a secret weapon: movement.

"It's not just about keeping your blood sugar in check," you explain, "though that's definitely a bonus! Think of exercise as a magic potion for your mind too."

Their eyes widen with curiosity. You continue, painting a vivid picture...

"Imagine your brain as a garden. Diabetes can be like a drought, leaving it parched and wilted. But exercise? It's like a refreshing rain shower. It nourishes those brain cells, helps them grow and flourish."

You describe how exercise unleashes a flood of feel-good chemicals like endorphins – natural mood boosters that create a sense of euphoria. It's like turning up the volume on your brain's happiness playlist.

"And it's not just a temporary fix," you assure them. "Exercise helps rewire your brain, making it more resilient to stress. Like building a strong fortress against those worries and anxieties."

You delve into the practical side, suggesting a mix of activities:

    Heart-pumping adventures: Brisk walks in nature, dancing like nobody's watching, or swimming in the sunlit pool.
    Strength training: Feeling the power surge through your muscles as you lift weights or use resistance bands.
    Mindful movement: Finding inner peace through yoga, tai chi, or meditation.

"The key is to find what you love," you emphasize, "something that makes you feel alive and joyful. It's not about pushing yourself to the limit, but about consistent, mindful movement."

You share inspiring stories of people who've transformed their lives through exercise:

    The woman who rediscovered her zest for life after joining a Zumba class.
    The man who found solace and strength in practicing yoga, taming his anxiety and improving his blood sugar control.

"It's a journey, not a race," you remind them. "Start small, listen to your body, and celebrate every step of the way. And remember, you're not alone. Talk to your doctor, find a supportive community, and embrace the power of movement to nurture both your body and mind."

As you finish, you see a spark of hope ignite in their eyes. They're ready to embark on this new adventure, armed with the knowledge that exercise is not just medicine for the body, but a potent elixir for the soul.

Subtopic 4: Integrating Exercise into Mental Health Care for Individuals with Diabetes

The Mind-Body Connection: How Exercise Can Empower Individuals with Diabetes and Mental Health Conditions

Living with diabetes can be a challenging journey, both physically and mentally. It's like walking a tightrope, constantly balancing blood sugar levels while navigating the emotional ups and downs that can come with the condition. But what if there was a tool that could help individuals with diabetes find more stability and resilience?

Enter exercise – a powerful ally that not only benefits physical health but also has a profound impact on mental well-being.

The Benefits of Exercise: A Holistic Approach to Well-being

Imagine exercise as a key that unlocks a treasure chest of benefits for individuals with diabetes and mental health conditions. This key opens the door to:

   Improved Glycemic Control: Like a conductor leading an orchestra, exercise helps harmonize blood sugar levels, making it easier to manage diabetes and reduce the risk of complications.
   Reduced Risk of Diabetes Complications: Think of exercise as a shield, protecting against the potential harms of diabetes, such as cardiovascular disease, nerve damage, and kidney problems.
   Mood Elevation and Reduced Symptoms of Depression and Anxiety: Exercise is like a natural mood booster, releasing endorphins that have a calming and uplifting effect on the mind.
   Increased Self-Esteem and Body Image: Engaging in physical activity can be a form of self-care, helping individuals feel more confident and comfortable in their own skin.
   Better Sleep Quality: Exercise is like a lullaby for the mind, promoting restful sleep and helping individuals wake up feeling refreshed and energized.
   Enhanced Cognitive Function: Like a brain workout, physical activity sharpens memory, attention, and decision-making abilities.

Integrating Exercise into Mental Health Treatment Plans: A Collaborative Approach

Integrating exercise into mental health treatment plans is like creating a personalized roadmap to well-being. It requires a collaborative effort between healthcare professionals, mental health professionals, and the individual with diabetes. Here are some key strategies:

Assessment and Individualized Exercise Prescription:

Comprehensive Assessment: Before embarking on an exercise journey, it's essential to take a holistic snapshot of the individual's physical and mental health. This includes understanding their diabetes management, current activity levels, exercise preferences, and any physical limitations.

Individualized Exercise Prescription: Just like a tailor creates a custom-made suit, healthcare professionals should design an exercise plan that fits the individual's unique needs and preferences. This plan should consider their fitness level, diabetes management goals, and mental health conditions, providing specific recommendations for frequency, intensity, duration, and type of exercise.

Goal Setting: Setting realistic and achievable exercise goals is like planting seeds of motivation. Breaking down larger goals into smaller, more manageable steps helps individuals experience a sense of accomplishment and progress.

Promoting Exercise Adherence:

Motivational Interviewing: Motivational interviewing is like a supportive conversation that helps individuals explore their ambivalence towards exercise, identify their personal values and goals, and find their own reasons for making a change.

Behavioral Activation: Behavioral activation is like a gentle nudge towards a more active lifestyle. It encourages individuals to gradually increase their activity levels by incorporating enjoyable activities into their daily routine, providing positive reinforcement and feedback along the way.

Problem-Solving and Skills Training: Equipping individuals with problem-solving skills is like giving them a toolkit to overcome barriers to exercise. Education on exercise safety, proper technique, and self-monitoring empowers them to take charge of their physical activity.

Social Support: Social support is like a cheering squad, providing encouragement and motivation. Connecting with family, friends, or support groups can make exercise more enjoyable and sustainable.

Technology-Assisted Interventions: Technology can be a valuable companion on the exercise journey. Wearable fitness trackers, mobile apps, and online resources can help individuals track their progress, receive feedback, and stay motivated.

Addressing Barriers to Exercise:

Physical Limitations: For individuals with physical limitations, working with a physical therapist or certified exercise professional is like having a guide to navigate the path to safe and effective exercise.

Lack of Time: Time management strategies are like finding hidden pockets of time in a busy schedule. Healthcare professionals can help individuals identify opportunities to incorporate exercise into their daily routine, such as taking short walks during breaks or using stairs instead of elevators.

Lack of Motivation: Addressing lack of motivation is like uncovering hidden treasures within. Exploring the individual's reasons for low motivation and addressing any underlying psychological barriers, such as depression or anxiety, can pave the way for a more active lifestyle.

Financial Constraints: Finding low-cost or free exercise options is like discovering hidden gems in the community. Healthcare professionals can provide information on community fitness programs, walking groups, or online exercise videos.

Fear of Hypoglycemia: Education on hypoglycemia prevention and management is like a safety net, empowering individuals to exercise with confidence. This includes adjusting medication dosages, monitoring blood sugar levels, and carrying snacks.

Collaborating with Mental Health Professionals:

Integrated Care Models: Integrated care models are like a symphony orchestra, with healthcare professionals, mental health professionals, and other relevant providers working together in harmony to provide comprehensive care.

Referral and Consultation: Referring individuals to mental health professionals is like seeking expert advice for specific needs. Consultation with mental health professionals on exercise recommendations and strategies to address psychological barriers can enhance the effectiveness of treatment plans.

Shared Decision-Making: Shared decision-making is like a collaborative dance, where healthcare professionals and individuals with diabetes work together to create a treatment plan that respects individual preferences and autonomy while providing evidence-based guidance.

Case Studies: Real-Life Examples of Transformation

Case Study 1: A 45-year-old woman with type 2 diabetes and depression finds new motivation for exercise through motivational interviewing and behavioral activation. She gradually increases her activity levels, improves her glycemic control, reduces her depressive symptoms, and enhances her overall quality of life.

Case Study 2: A 60-year-old man with type 1 diabetes and anxiety overcomes physical limitations and financial constraints with the help of a physical therapist and information on low-cost exercise options. He improves his physical function, increases his exercise participation, reduces his anxiety symptoms, and achieves better diabetes management.

Conclusion: Empowering Individuals with Diabetes and Mental Health Conditions through Exercise

Integrating exercise into mental health care for individuals with diabetes is like giving them a superpower to transform their lives. By utilizing evidence-based strategies, addressing barriers, and collaborating with mental health professionals, healthcare providers can empower individuals with diabetes to embrace an active lifestyle, leading to better diabetes management, improved mental health, and a more fulfilling life.

Exercise and Sleep: A Synergistic Duo for Diabetes Management

The Silent Thief of Slumber: How Sleep Disorders Sabotage Your Metabolism

Imagine your body as a bustling city at night. While you sleep, intricate repair crews are hard at work, regulating energy, balancing hormones, and keeping everything running smoothly. But what happens when those crews are constantly interrupted by noisy neighbors, roadblocks, or flickering traffic lights? Chaos ensues, and in the case of your body, that chaos manifests as metabolic dysregulation.

Sleep disorders, those pesky villains of the night, are like those disruptive neighbors, wreaking havoc on your metabolic health. Let's shine a light on some of the worst offenders:

Insomnia: The Wide-Eyed Worrywart: Insomnia is like a relentless alarm clock in your mind, keeping you awake and your stress hormones soaring. Cortisol, the body's main stress hormone, becomes your metabolic enemy, flooding your system and making it harder for your cells to use energy efficiently. Think of it as cortisol turning up the sugar production in your body while simultaneously locking the doors to your muscles, preventing them from using that sugar. The result? A recipe for high blood sugar and insulin resistance.

Obstructive Sleep Apnea (OSA): The Nighttime Choker: OSA is like a mischievous gremlin that sneaks in while you sleep and intermittently cuts off your oxygen supply. Your body, in a panic, sends out stress signals, further disrupting your metabolism. It's like trying to run a marathon while constantly gasping for air – your body just can't keep up.

Circadian Rhythm Disruptions: The Time-Traveling Troublemaker: Our bodies operate on a 24-hour internal clock, dictating when we sleep, wake, and perform various metabolic functions. Circadian rhythm disruptions are like throwing a wrench in that clock, causing your body's internal timing to go haywire. Hormones become unbalanced, and your metabolism is left scrambling to catch up.

The Vicious Cycle of Sleeplessness, Weight Gain, and Diabetes

Sleep disorders, obesity, and diabetes often form an unwelcome trio, each exacerbating the other. It's like a three-way tug-of-war, with your health caught in the middle. Obesity increases your risk of developing OSA, while OSA can worsen insulin resistance and promote weight gain. This creates a vicious cycle that can be difficult to break.

What Can You Do?

The good news is that you don't have to surrender to these sleep saboteurs. Here are some strategies to reclaim your sleep and protect your metabolic health:

Prioritize Sleep Hygiene: Make sleep a non-negotiable part of your routine. Create a relaxing bedtime ritual, avoid caffeine and alcohol before bed, and keep your bedroom cool, dark, and quiet.
Seek Professional Help: If you suspect you have a sleep disorder, don't hesitate to consult a healthcare professional. There are effective treatments available,

ranging from lifestyle modifications to CPAP therapy for OSA.

Manage Stress: Stress is a major contributor to sleep problems. Find healthy ways to manage stress, such as exercise, yoga, meditation, or spending time in nature.

Remember, sleep is not a luxury; it's a necessity for a healthy metabolism. By prioritizing sleep and addressing any underlying sleep disorders, you can take a significant step towards improving your metabolic health and overall well-being.

Sweet Dreams: How Exercise Can Improve Sleep for People with Diabetes

Sleepless nights plague many people with diabetes, but there's a powerful remedy that doesn't involve pills or potions – exercise!

The Sleep-Diabetes Connection

Diabetes can disrupt your sleep in a number of ways. High blood sugar levels can interfere with the body's natural sleep-wake cycle, leading to trouble falling asleep, frequent awakenings during the night, and early morning wake-ups. This sleep deprivation can, in turn, worsen your diabetes control, creating a vicious cycle.

Exercise to the Rescue

Regular physical activity is a natural sleep enhancer that can significantly improve sleep quality for people with diabetes. Here's how it works:

Regulating the Body's Clock: Exercise helps regulate your circadian rhythm, the body's internal clock that controls sleep-wake patterns. It does this by increasing the production of melatonin, a hormone that promotes sleep.

Stress Reduction: Exercise can help reduce stress levels, which can interfere with sleep. It releases endorphins, the body's natural feel-good hormones, promoting relaxation and creating a more conducive environment for sleep.

Better Sleep Architecture: Exercise can improve the quality of your sleep by increasing the amount of deep sleep and REM sleep, both of which are essential for physical and mental well-being.

Research Says It Works!

Numerous studies have shown that exercise can significantly improve sleep quality in people with diabetes. Some studies have found that exercise can increase total sleep time, reduce the time it takes to fall asleep, and decrease the number of nighttime awakenings. Other studies have shown that exercise can improve sleep efficiency, the percentage of time spent asleep once you're in bed.

Types of Exercise that Help

Most types of exercise can improve sleep, but some may be more beneficial than others. Moderate-intensity aerobic exercise, such as brisk walking, jogging, cycling, or swimming, is generally recommended. Strength training can also be helpful, especially for people with type 2 diabetes.

How Much Exercise is Enough?

Aim for at least 150 minutes of moderate-intensity aerobic exercise per week, spread throughout the week. You can also break it up into shorter sessions, such as 30 minutes of exercise five days a week.

Tips for Better Sleep

In addition to exercise, there are a few other things you can do to improve your sleep quality:

   Establish a regular sleep schedule: Go to bed and wake up at the same time each day, even on weekends.
   Create a relaxing bedtime routine: 1 Take a warm bath, read a book, or listen to calming music before bed.
   Make sure your bedroom is dark, quiet, and cool: A comfortable sleep environment is essential for good sleep.
   Avoid caffeine and alcohol before bed: Caffeine and alcohol can interfere with sleep.
   Limit screen time before bed: The blue light from screens can suppress melatonin production and make it harder to fall asleep.

Talk to Your Doctor

If you have diabetes and are having trouble sleeping, talk to your doctor. They can help you develop a safe and effective exercise plan that's right for you.

Sweet Dreams!

By making exercise a part of your daily routine, you can improve your sleep quality, manage your diabetes better, and feel your best.

Sweet Dreams: The Key to Better Blood Sugar Control

Drifting off into a deep, restful sleep might sound like a luxury, but for people with diabetes, it's actually a vital part of managing their condition. Good sleep plays a crucial role in regulating blood sugar levels, keeping insulin resistance in check, and reducing the risk of complications. Think of it as the body's natural way to recharge and reset, and when it's disrupted, things can go awry.

The Sleep-Diabetes Connection

It's a two-way street: poor sleep can mess with blood sugar, and diabetes itself can make it harder to get a good night's rest. When you don't get enough sleep, your body produces more of the stress hormone cortisol, which can raise blood sugar levels. Plus, sleep deprivation can make your cells less responsive to insulin, the hormone that helps move sugar into your cells for energy.

On the other hand, diabetes can lead to conditions that disrupt sleep. For example, high blood sugar can cause frequent urination and thirst, making it hard to fall asleep and stay asleep. Other complications like nerve damage (neuropathy) or restless legs syndrome can also keep you up at night.

Sweet Dreams: How to Optimize Your Sleep

Establish a Regular Sleep Schedule: Go to bed and wake up at the same time each day, even on weekends. This helps regulate your body's internal clock and makes it easier to fall asleep and stay asleep.

2. **Create a Relaxing Bedtime Routine:** Wind down before bed with activities that help you relax, like taking a warm bath, reading a book, or listening to calming music. Avoid screens for at least an hour before bed, as the blue light they emit can disrupt your sleep-wake cycle.

Optimize Your Sleep Environment: Make sure your bedroom is dark, quiet, and cool. Invest in a comfortable mattress and pillows, and create a clutter-free environment that promotes relaxation.

Address Underlying Sleep Disorders: If you snore, have trouble breathing during sleep, or experience restless legs syndrome, talk to your doctor. These conditions can disrupt sleep and worsen diabetes control.

Manage Your Stress Levels: Stress can interfere with sleep, so find healthy ways to manage it, such as exercise, meditation, or spending time in nature.

Watch Your Diet and Exercise: Eating a healthy diet and getting regular exercise can also improve your sleep quality. Aim for a balanced diet that's low in processed foods and sugary drinks, and choose moderate-intensity exercise most days of the week.

Remember, everyone's sleep needs are different. If you're having trouble sleeping, don't hesitate to talk to your doctor. They can help you identify any underlying causes and develop a personalized plan to improve your sleep quality.

By prioritizing sleep, you can take a significant step towards better blood sugar control and overall well-being. Sweet dreams!

Sweet Dreams and Sweaty Success: A Guide to Integrating Exercise and Sleep for Diabetes Management

Introduction

In the realm of diabetes management, a growing body of evidence underscores the crucial role of both exercise and sleep in regulating blood sugar levels, improving overall health, and reducing the risk of complications. This comprehensive guide delves into the synergistic interplay between exercise, sleep, and diabetes, offering practical guidance for healthcare professionals to integrate these interventions into their clinical practice.

Understanding the Sweet Symphony: Exercise, Sleep, and Diabetes

Imagine exercise and sleep as two powerful instruments, each playing a unique tune in the symphony of diabetes management. When played in harmony, they create a beautiful melody that can significantly improve glycemic control, weight management, cardiovascular health, and mental well-being.

The Power of Synergy

Improved Insulin Sensitivity: Both exercise and adequate sleep enhance insulin sensitivity, a key factor in regulating blood sugar levels. Exercise increases glucose uptake by muscles, while sleep promotes hormonal balance crucial for insulin action. Combining these interventions can lead to significant improvements in glycemic control.

Weight Management: Regular physical activity and sufficient sleep contribute to weight loss or maintenance, which is essential for diabetes management. Sleep deprivation can disrupt appetite-regulating hormones, leading to increased food cravings and weight gain.

Reduced Cardiovascular Risk: Exercise and sleep play vital roles in cardiovascular health, a major concern for individuals with diabetes. Exercise strengthens the heart and improves circulation, while sleep allows for repair and recovery. Addressing both factors can significantly reduce the risk of heart disease, stroke, and other complications.

Enhanced Mental Well-being: Diabetes management can be emotionally challenging. Exercise and sleep both positively impact mental health by reducing stress, improving mood, and enhancing cognitive function. Integrating these interventions can contribute to better overall well-being and improve adherence to diabetes management plans.

The Bidirectional Dance

Exercise and sleep are not independent entities but interact in a complex bidirectional relationship. Regular physical activity generally promotes better sleep quality, but excessive exercise close to bedtime can interfere with sleep. Similarly, poor sleep can reduce motivation to exercise and impair physical performance.

Sleep deprivation can negatively impact glucose metabolism, leading to insulin resistance and elevated blood sugar levels. Conversely, poor glycemic control can disrupt sleep patterns, causing frequent awakenings and reduced sleep quality. Understanding this complex interplay is crucial for developing effective, personalized interventions.

A Practical Guide for Healthcare Professionals

Comprehensive Assessment

To provide optimal care, healthcare professionals should conduct a comprehensive assessment of each patient's individual needs and preferences. This includes:

Detailed Medical History: Gather information on the patient's diabetes type, duration, current medications, comorbidities, and any sleep disorders.
Sleep Evaluation: Assess sleep quality and duration using tools like the Pittsburgh Sleep Quality Index (PSQI) or actigraphy. Identify any sleep disturbances, such as insomnia, sleep apnea, or restless legs syndrome.
Physical Activity Assessment: Evaluate current physical activity levels, exercise preferences, and any limitations or contraindications. Consider using questionnaires or wearable devices to track activity patterns.

Personalized Intervention Strategies

Based on the assessment findings, healthcare professionals can develop personalized intervention strategies that address both exercise and sleep.

Tailored Exercise Prescriptions:
Type: Recommend aerobic exercises (e.g., brisk walking, swimming, cycling), resistance training (e.g., weightlifting, bodyweight exercises), and flexibility exercises (e.g., yoga, stretching) based on individual needs and preferences.
Intensity: Start with moderate-intensity activities and gradually increase intensity and duration as fitness improves. Monitor blood glucose levels before, during, and after exercise to adjust intensity as needed.

Frequency: Aim for at least 150 minutes of moderate-intensity or 75 minutes of vigorous-intensity aerobic activity per week, spread throughout the week. Encourage resistance training 2-3 times per week.

Timing: Consider the timing of exercise in relation to meals and medication to optimize glycemic control. Advise against vigorous exercise close to bedtime.

Sleep Optimization Strategies:

Sleep Hygiene Education: Provide guidance on creating a conducive sleep environment, establishing a regular sleep schedule, and practicing relaxing bedtime routines.

Cognitive Behavioral Therapy for Insomnia (CBT-I): If insomnia is present, consider referral to a sleep specialist for CBT-I, a highly effective treatment for chronic insomnia.

Addressing Sleep Disorders: Screen for and manage sleep disorders like sleep apnea, restless legs syndrome, and circadian rhythm disorders.

Medication Review: Evaluate medications that may interfere with sleep and adjust dosages or timings as appropriate.

An Integrated Approach

Combining exercise and sleep interventions is more than just the sum of its parts. It's about creating a synergistic effect that can lead to even greater improvements in health outcomes.

Comprehensive Plan: Develop a comprehensive plan that addresses both exercise and sleep, emphasizing the synergistic benefits of both.

Patient-Centered Approach: Involve patients in decision-making, considering their preferences, lifestyle, and individual needs.

Gradual Implementation: Encourage gradual changes in exercise and sleep habits to promote long-term adherence.

   Regular Monitoring and Follow-up: Monitor progress regularly, adjust interventions as needed, and provide ongoing support and motivation.

The Role of Technology

In today's digital age, technology can be a powerful ally in the integration of exercise and sleep interventions.

   Wearable Devices: Utilize fitness trackers and smartwatches to monitor activity levels, sleep patterns, and heart rate. This data can provide valuable insights for personalized recommendations and progress tracking.

   Mobile Apps: Employ apps that offer exercise guidance, sleep tracking, and diabetes management tools to enhance self-management and provide educational resources.

   Telehealth: Utilize telehealth platforms for remote monitoring, consultations, and support, particularly for patients with limited access to in-person care.

Case Studies

To illustrate the effectiveness of integrated exercise and sleep interventions, let's consider two real-life examples:

   Mr. A, a 55-year-old man with type 2 diabetes: Mr. A struggled with poorly controlled blood sugar levels, a sedentary lifestyle, and sleep difficulties. Through a combination of exercise prescription, sleep hygiene education, and sleep apnea treatment, he achieved significant improvements in his blood sugar control, weight loss, sleep quality, and overall well-being.

Ms. B, a 30-year-old woman with type 1 diabetes: Ms. B experienced fluctuating blood sugar levels, anxiety, and irregular sleep patterns due to a demanding work schedule. By incorporating high-intensity interval training, yoga, mindfulness practices, and sleep hygiene education, she was able to improve her glycemic control, reduce anxiety levels, and achieve more consistent sleep patterns.

Long-Term Follow-up and Maintenance

Integrating exercise and sleep interventions is not a one-time event but rather a lifelong commitment. Healthcare professionals play a crucial role in providing ongoing support and motivation to ensure long-term adherence and success.

Ongoing Support: Provide continued support and encouragement through regular check-ups, phone calls, or online platforms.
Reinforcement and Motivation: Reinforce the importance of maintaining healthy habits and address any challenges or setbacks.
Adaptation and Adjustment: Adjust interventions as needed based on individual progress, lifestyle changes, and evolving health needs.
Group Support: Consider offering group programs or support groups to foster peer support and motivation.

Research Focus

The field of exercise and sleep interventions for diabetes management is constantly evolving. Ongoing research is crucial to:

Multimodal Interventions: Evaluate the effectiveness of multimodal interventions that combine exercise, sleep optimization, dietary modifications, and stress management for achieving long-term diabetes management success.

Patient-Centered Approaches: Investigate the impact of patient-centered approaches on adherence, outcomes, and quality of life.

Long-Term Follow-up Studies: Conduct long-term follow-up studies to assess the sustainability of behavior changes and the long-term impact of integrated interventions.

Conclusion

Integrating exercise and sleep interventions is essential for comprehensive diabetes management. Healthcare professionals play a crucial role in educating patients, providing personalized guidance, and offering ongoing support. By adopting a multimodal, patient-centered approach and staying abreast of the latest research, healthcare professionals can empower individuals with diabetes to achieve optimal glycemic control, improve overall health, and reduce the risk of complications.

Remember, a healthy lifestyle is the cornerstone of diabetes management. By integrating exercise and sleep into their daily routine, individuals with diabetes can take control of their health and lead fulfilling lives.

Let's work together to create a healthier future for people with diabetes!

Exercise Prescription for the Aging Population with Diabetes

The "Use It or Lose It" Years: Why Exercise Matters More Than Ever

Let's face it, getting older isn't always a picnic. Our bodies change, things start to creak a bit, and suddenly that morning jog feels more like a marathon. And if you're living with diabetes, well, that adds another layer of complexity to the mix.

But here's the good news: aging doesn't have to mean slowing down. In fact, staying active is one of the most powerful things you can do to live a longer, healthier, and more vibrant life, especially with diabetes.

Think of your body like a classic car. With proper care and maintenance, that vintage beauty can keep running smoothly for decades. But neglect it, and it'll start to rust, sputter, and eventually break down. Exercise is like the tune-up your body needs to stay in top shape.
What Happens When the "Check Engine" Light Comes On?

As we age, our bodies go through some natural changes. It's like the "check engine" light flashing on your dashboard – a signal that things need a little attention. Here are a few of the common "alerts" you might experience:

   Muscle Meltdown (Sarcopenia): Imagine your muscles as a vibrant garden. Without regular tending, those beautiful blooms start to wither and fade. Sarcopenia, or age-related muscle loss, is a bit like that. Diabetes can speed up this process, making it even more important to "fertilize" your muscles with regular strength training.

Bone Brittle (Osteoporosis): Think of your bones as the sturdy frame of that classic car. Over time, they can become thinner and weaker, especially for women. Diabetes can accelerate this process, increasing the risk of fractures. But just like reinforcing the chassis of a car, weight-bearing exercises and a calcium-rich diet can help keep your bones strong and resilient.

Engine Trouble (Cardiovascular Changes): Your heart is the engine that keeps everything running. As we age, this mighty pump can lose some of its horsepower. Diabetes can add to the strain, increasing the risk of heart disease. But aerobic exercise is like a high-octane fuel that keeps your heart pumping strong and your blood flowing smoothly.

Fuel System Glitches (Metabolic Changes): Just like a car needs the right fuel to run efficiently, your body needs glucose to function properly. Aging and diabetes can make it harder for your body to use this fuel effectively, leading to high blood sugar. But regular exercise can help improve your body's "fuel efficiency" and keep your blood sugar in check.

Stay tuned for Part 2, where we'll explore how to customize your exercise plan and keep your body running like a well-oiled machine!

What's different here?

Engaging language: I've used metaphors (classic car, garden, engine) to make the information more relatable and memorable.

Conversational tone: The writing is more informal and friendly, like a conversation with a friend.

Positive framing: The focus is on empowerment and the potential for positive change, rather than just listing problems.

Cliffhanger: Ending with a "stay tuned" creates anticipation and encourages readers to continue learning.

This is just one example, of course. I can continue to apply these principles to the rest of your review, creating a truly unique and engaging piece that resonates with your audience. Let me know what you think!

Exercise: Your Prescription for a Healthier Life with Diabetes

Diabetes is a chronic condition that affects millions of people worldwide. It's characterized by high blood sugar levels, which can lead to a range of health problems, including heart disease, stroke, kidney disease, and nerve damage. While managing diabetes can be challenging, regular exercise is a powerful tool that can significantly improve your health and well-being.

Benefits of Exercise for People with Diabetes

Improved Blood Sugar Control: Exercise helps your body use insulin more effectively, lowering your blood sugar levels. It also helps prevent spikes in blood sugar after meals.

Reduced Risk of Complications: Regular exercise can lower your risk of developing serious diabetes-related complications, such as heart disease, stroke, and kidney disease.

Weight Management: Maintaining a healthy weight is important for people with diabetes. Exercise can help you lose weight or maintain a healthy weight, which can improve your blood sugar control and overall health.

Improved Cardiovascular Health: Exercise strengthens your heart and lungs, reducing your risk of heart disease and improving your cardiovascular health.

Enhanced Mental Health: Exercise can help reduce stress, anxiety, and depression, which are common among people with diabetes.

Improved Quality of Life: Exercise can help you feel better physically and emotionally, leading to an improved overall quality of life.

Types of Exercise

There are many different types of exercise that are beneficial for people with diabetes. Some of the best options include:

Aerobic exercise: Aerobic exercise is any activity that raises your heart rate and breathing. Examples include walking, jogging, swimming, cycling, and dancing. Aim for at least 150 minutes of moderate-intensity aerobic exercise or 75 minutes of vigorous-intensity aerobic exercise per week.

Resistance training: Resistance training is any activity that builds muscle strength. Examples include lifting weights, using resistance bands, or doing calisthenics. Aim for at least two days of resistance training per week.

Flexibility exercises: Flexibility exercises help to improve your range of motion and prevent injuries. Examples include stretching, yoga, and Pilates.

Tips for Getting Started

Start slowly and gradually increase the intensity and duration of your workouts.
Choose activities that you enjoy and that 1 fit your fitness level.
Find a workout buddy or join a fitness class to help you stay motivated.
Talk to your doctor before starting any new exercise program.

Additional Considerations

Check your blood sugar before and after exercise.
Be aware of the signs of low blood sugar, such as sweating, dizziness, and confusion.
Carry snacks or drinks with you to prevent low blood sugar.
Wear comfortable clothing and shoes.
Warm up and cool down before and after exercise.
Listen to your body and rest if you feel tired or sore.

Making Exercise a Part of Your Life

Exercise is an important part of a healthy lifestyle for everyone, including people with diabetes. By making exercise a regular part of your routine, you can improve your blood sugar control, reduce your risk of complications, and enjoy a better quality of life.

Tailoring Exercise Programs for Older Adults with Diabetes: A Guide to Safe and Effective Fitness

Diabetes is a common and serious chronic condition that affects millions of people worldwide. While it can be challenging to manage, regular exercise is a crucial part of a healthy lifestyle for individuals with diabetes. It can help improve blood sugar control, lower the risk of complications, and enhance overall well-being. However, designing exercise programs for older adults with diabetes requires careful consideration of their unique needs and limitations.

This guide will provide evidence-based recommendations for tailoring exercise programs to optimize safety and effectiveness in older adults with diabetes. We will discuss key considerations such as individual assessment, exercise prescription guidelines, safety considerations, adapted physical activity programs, comorbidities and functional limitations, and preferences and motivation.

Key Considerations for Exercise Prescription in Older Adults with Diabetes

Individualized Assessment: A comprehensive assessment is essential to gather information about an individual's medical history, current health status, functional capacity, and any existing comorbidities. This assessment should include:

Medical History: Diabetes type and management, medications, history of hypoglycemia or hyperglycemia, cardiovascular disease risk factors, other chronic conditions.
Functional Capacity: Assess physical function using tools like the Senior Fitness Test, Timed Up and Go test, and gait speed assessment.
Cognitive Status: Evaluate cognitive function using tools like the Mini-Mental State Examination (MMSE) or Montreal Cognitive Assessment (MoCA) to identify any cognitive impairment that may affect exercise participation.
Nutritional Status: Assess dietary habits and nutritional status to identify any potential risks or deficiencies that may impact exercise tolerance.

Psychosocial Factors: Evaluate social support, motivation, and any psychological barriers to exercise participation.

Exercise Prescription Guidelines:

Aerobic Exercise:
Frequency: At least 150 minutes of moderate-intensity or 75 minutes of vigorous-intensity aerobic exercise per week, spread throughout the week.
Intensity: Moderate-intensity exercise is recommended for most older adults with diabetes. Use the talk test or Borg Rating of Perceived Exertion (RPE) scale to monitor intensity.
Type: Encourage activities that are enjoyable and accessible, such as walking, swimming, cycling, dancing, or water aerobics.
Progression: Gradually increase exercise duration and intensity as tolerated.

Resistance Training:
Frequency: At least 2-3 days per week, targeting major muscle groups.
Intensity: Start with light to moderate intensity and gradually increase as strength improves. Use the RPE scale to monitor intensity.
Type: Include exercises that use body weight, resistance bands, or light weights.
Repetitions and Sets: Aim for 8-12 repetitions for each exercise and 1-3 sets per muscle group.

Flexibility and Balance Exercises:
Frequency: At least 2-3 days per week.
Type: Include static stretches, dynamic stretches, and balance exercises such as yoga, tai chi, or Pilates.
Duration: Hold each stretch for 15-30 seconds and repeat 2-4 times.

Safety Considerations:

Blood Glucose Monitoring: Monitor blood glucose levels before, during, and after exercise, especially when starting a new exercise program or changing intensity or duration.
Hydration: Drink plenty of fluids before, during, and after exercise to prevent dehydration.
Foot Care: Wear proper footwear and inspect feet regularly for any signs of injury or infection.
Environmental Factors: Consider exercising in a safe and comfortable environment, especially during extreme weather conditions.
Medical Clearance: Consult with a healthcare provider before starting any new exercise program, especially if there are any underlying health conditions or concerns.

Adapted Physical Activity Programs:

Chair Exercises: For older adults with limited mobility or balance issues, chair exercises can provide a safe and effective way to improve strength, flexibility, and cardiovascular health.
Aquatic Exercise: Water provides buoyancy and support, making it an ideal exercise modality for older adults with joint pain or arthritis.
Yoga and Tai Chi: These mind-body practices can improve balance, flexibility, and reduce stress.
Walking Programs: Structured walking programs can be tailored to individual fitness levels and preferences.

Comorbidities and Functional Limitations:

Arthritis: Modify exercises to reduce joint stress and pain. Consider low-impact activities like swimming or cycling.
Cardiovascular Disease: Monitor heart rate and blood pressure closely during exercise. Start with low-intensity activities and gradually increase as tolerated.

Neuropathy: Wear proper footwear and avoid high-impact activities that may increase the risk of foot injury.

Cognitive Impairment: Provide clear and simple instructions, use visual cues, and offer frequent encouragement and support.

Preferences and Motivation:

Enjoyable Activities: Encourage older adults to choose activities they enjoy and are likely to stick with.

Social Support: Group exercise classes or exercising with a friend or family member can provide motivation and support.

Goal Setting: Help older adults set realistic and achievable exercise goals.

Positive Reinforcement: Provide positive feedback and encouragement to promote adherence to the exercise program.

Case Studies

Case Study 1:

Patient: 70-year-old female with type 2 diabetes, osteoarthritis, and mild cognitive impairment.

Assessment: Limited mobility due to knee pain, decreased balance, and difficulty following complex instructions.

Exercise Program:

Chair exercises 3 times per week, focusing on strengthening major muscle groups and improving range of motion.

Aquatic exercise 2 times per week, including walking in the pool and water aerobics.

Balance exercises daily, including standing on one leg and heel-toe walking.

Simple yoga poses for flexibility and relaxation.

Case Study 2:

Patient: 80-year-old male with type 2 diabetes, peripheral neuropathy, and history of falls.
Assessment: Decreased sensation in feet, impaired balance, and fear of falling.
Exercise Program:
Tai chi 2 times per week to improve balance and coordination.
Walking program 3 times per week, starting with short distances and gradually increasing duration.
Resistance training 2 times per week, focusing on upper body strength and core stability.
Foot care education and regular foot inspections.

Conclusion

Tailoring exercise programs for older adults with diabetes requires a comprehensive and individualized approach. By considering individual needs, functional limitations, comorbidities, and preferences, healthcare professionals can design safe and effective exercise programs that promote health, well-being, and successful diabetes management. Regular exercise can help older adults with diabetes improve their cardiovascular health, manage blood glucose levels, maintain a healthy weight, enhance functional capacity, and reduce the risk of complications. By empowering older adults with diabetes to engage in regular physical activity, we can support them in living longer, healthier, and more fulfilling lives.

Additional Resources

American Diabetes Association: https://www.diabetes.org/
American College of Sports Medicine: https://www.acsm.org/

World Health Organization: https://www.who.int/
National Institute on Aging: https://www.nia.nih.gov/

Note: This information is intended for educational purposes only and should not be considered medical advice. Always consult with a qualified healthcare professional before starting any new exercise program.

Stepping into Stride: Empowering Older Adults with Diabetes to Embrace Movement

Imagine a life where your golden years are truly golden – filled with energy, vitality, and the freedom to live life to the fullest. For older adults with diabetes, exercise isn't just a recommendation, it's a lifeline. It's the key to managing blood sugar, keeping those hearts strong, and boosting overall well-being. But let's face it, getting started and staying motivated can be a challenge.

The Hurdles on the Path to Fitness

Before we jump into solutions, let's acknowledge the real-life hurdles that many older adults with diabetes face:

Fear of Falling: The fear of taking a tumble can be a major roadblock, especially for those with diabetes-related complications like neuropathy or vision problems.
Pain as a Barrier: Chronic pain from conditions like arthritis or diabetic neuropathy can make exercise feel like an uphill battle.
Motivation Malaise: It's tough to find the get-up-and-go when facing health challenges or competing priorities.
Lonely Workouts: Lack of support from family, friends, or healthcare providers can make exercise feel isolating.
Access Denied: Limited transportation, financial constraints, or lack of accessible facilities can create frustrating obstacles.

Blood Sugar Worries: Concerns about hypoglycemia (low blood sugar) during or after exercise can be a real deterrent.

Turning Challenges into Triumphs: Strategies for Success

Let's explore how we can transform these challenges into opportunities for a healthier, more active life:

1. Conquering the Fear of Falling:

   Personalized Plans: Imagine exercise programs tailored to individual fitness levels, balance abilities, and health conditions. Think low-impact activities like tai chi, swimming, or walking, gradually increasing in intensity and duration.
   Balance Boosters: Incorporating balance-enhancing exercises like single-leg stances, heel-toe walks, and standing on unstable surfaces can help build confidence and reduce fall risk.
   Strength for Stability: Building muscle strength through resistance exercises using body weight, bands, or light weights can significantly improve stability.
   Safe and Sound Environments: Creating a safe exercise space by removing tripping hazards, ensuring adequate lighting, and using assistive devices like canes or walkers when needed is crucial.
   Knowledge is Power: Educating older adults about fall prevention strategies and addressing their fears through counseling can empower them to exercise safely.

2. Managing Pain, Maximizing Movement:

   Pain Relief Strategies: Working with healthcare providers to optimize pain management through medications, physical therapy, or alternative therapies can make exercise more comfortable.

Exercise Modifications: Adapting exercises to accommodate pain levels by choosing low-impact activities, reducing intensity or duration, or using modifications like chairs or supports is essential.

Understanding Pain: Educating older adults about the positive relationship between exercise and pain can help them understand that appropriate physical activity can actually reduce pain in the long run.

Mind-Body Connection: Practices like yoga, tai chi, and meditation can help manage pain, reduce stress, and improve overall well-being, making exercise more enjoyable.

3. Building a Support System for Success:

Group Power: Participating in group exercise classes can provide social interaction, encouragement, and accountability, making exercise more enjoyable and motivating.

Workout Buddies: Pairing older adults with exercise buddies can provide support, companionship, and motivation.

Family and Friends as Cheerleaders: Encouraging family members and caregivers to support and participate in exercise can enhance adherence.

Community Connections: Connecting older adults with community-based programs that offer exercise classes, social activities, and resources can foster a supportive environment.

4. Finding the Fun in Fitness:

Personalized Preferences: Tailoring exercise recommendations to individual interests and preferences is crucial for promoting adherence. This may involve exploring various activities like dancing, gardening, swimming, or cycling.

Goal Setting for Success: Setting realistic and achievable exercise goals can enhance motivation and provide a sense of accomplishment.

Positive Reinforcement: Providing positive feedback and encouragement can help older adults stay motivated and build confidence.

Technology as a Tool: Using technology like fitness trackers, mobile apps, or virtual exercise programs can enhance engagement and provide feedback.

Behavioral Interventions and Motivational Interviewing:

Motivational Interviewing: This counseling technique helps individuals explore their ambivalence about behavior change and identify their own motivations for exercise. It focuses on empowering individuals to make informed decisions and set realistic goals.

Cognitive-Behavioral Therapy (CBT): CBT can help address negative thoughts and beliefs that hinder exercise adherence. It focuses on developing coping strategies and building self-efficacy.

Problem-Solving Therapy: This approach helps individuals identify and overcome barriers to exercise by developing practical solutions.

Relapse Prevention: Strategies for preventing relapse and maintaining long-term adherence are essential. This may involve identifying triggers, developing coping mechanisms, and setting up support systems.

Community-Based Programs: A Hub for Healthy Living:

Community-based programs play a vital role in promoting exercise adherence among older adults with diabetes. These programs can provide:

Accessible and Affordable Exercise Classes: Offering a variety of classes tailored to different fitness levels and preferences, with options for low-impact activities and modifications for those with limitations.

Social Support and Interaction: Creating a welcoming and supportive environment where participants can connect with others and build relationships.

Education and Resources: Providing information about diabetes management, exercise benefits, and healthy lifestyle choices.

Trained Instructors: Ensuring that instructors are knowledgeable about diabetes and aging and can provide safe and effective exercise guidance.

Real-Life Success Stories:

Case Study 1: A 70-year-old woman with type 2 diabetes and osteoarthritis was hesitant to exercise due to knee pain and fear of falling. Through a community-based program, she discovered the joy of water aerobics. The low-impact environment and social support helped her gain confidence, reduce pain, and improve her blood sugar control.

Case Study 2: A 65-year-old man with type 2 diabetes and a history of heart disease was initially reluctant to exercise. Through a cardiac rehabilitation program that incorporated motivational interviewing, he was able to overcome his hesitation, adopt a regular exercise routine, and improve both his cardiovascular health and diabetes management.

Conclusion: Embracing Movement, Embracing Life

Promoting exercise adherence in older adults with diabetes requires a holistic approach that addresses individual barriers, provides social support, and promotes enjoyable physical activities. By utilizing evidence-based strategies like motivational interviewing, behavioral interventions, and community-based programs, healthcare providers can empower older adults to embrace an active lifestyle, leading to improved health outcomes and a more fulfilling life.

Combating the Rise of Type 2 Diabetes in Youth Through Exercise

The Pediatric Diabetes Epidemic: A Looming Crisis and a Call to Action

A Generation at Risk: The Alarming Rise of Type 2 Diabetes in Children

Imagine a world where our children, instead of brimming with energy and vitality, are burdened with a disease that was once considered an adult concern. This is the stark reality we face today as type 2 diabetes (T2DM), a condition historically associated with aging and unhealthy lifestyles, is increasingly encroaching upon the lives of our young people.

This isn't just a medical issue; it's a societal crisis. The "pediatric diabetes epidemic," as it's now known, is a wake-up call, a stark reminder of the urgent need to protect the health of our future generations.

Unmasking the Enemy: Understanding the Risk Factors

The rise of T2DM in children and adolescents is a complex issue, fueled by a confluence of factors. While genetics play a role, lifestyle choices are increasingly recognized as major culprits.

    The Obesity Crisis: The link between obesity and T2DM is undeniable. Excess body fat, especially around the abdomen, disrupts the body's ability to use insulin effectively, leading to a dangerous buildup of sugar in the blood.
    The Inactivity Trap: Our modern world, with its screens and sedentary lifestyles, has created an environment

where physical activity is often an afterthought. This lack of movement further exacerbates the risk of T2DM.

The Family Connection: Children with a family history of T2DM are at a significantly higher risk of developing the disease themselves. This highlights the importance of family-wide interventions to promote healthy habits.

The Dietary Dilemma: The prevalence of processed foods, sugary drinks, and unhealthy fats in our diets has created a nutritional minefield for our children. These dietary choices contribute to weight gain and insulin resistance, setting the stage for T2DM.

Turning the Tide: Prevention Strategies for a Healthier Future

The good news is that T2DM is largely preventable. By addressing the risk factors head-on, we can empower our children to live healthier lives.

Nourishing Our Children: Promoting healthy eating habits is paramount. This means encouraging the consumption of whole foods, fruits, vegetables, and lean protein while limiting processed foods, sugary drinks, and unhealthy fats.

Getting Kids Moving: Regular physical activity is crucial for maintaining a healthy weight and improving insulin sensitivity. We need to create environments where physical activity is encouraged and accessible.

Tackling Obesity: Addressing the obesity epidemic is a cornerstone of T2DM prevention. This requires a multi-pronged approach, including promoting healthy eating habits, encouraging physical activity, and creating supportive environments.

Empowering Families: Family-based interventions can be highly effective in promoting healthy lifestyles. Educating families about healthy habits and providing support for behavior change can make a significant difference.

Public Health in Action: Public health initiatives play a vital role in T2DM prevention. This includes policies that promote healthy food choices, create supportive environments for physical activity, and increase access to healthcare services.

Case Studies: Real-Life Stories, Real-Life Solutions

A Wake-Up Call: A 12-year-old boy, struggling with fatigue and excessive thirst, is diagnosed with T2DM. His family history and weight issues paint a clear picture of the challenges he faces. Lifestyle modifications, including dietary changes and increased physical activity, become his lifeline.

A Success Story: A 15-year-old girl, determined to break the cycle of T2DM in her family, joins a community-based program focused on healthy living. Through education, support, and resources, she transforms her habits and reduces her risk of developing the disease.

Conclusion: A Call to Action

The pediatric diabetes epidemic is a complex issue, but it's not insurmountable. By working together – parents, educators, healthcare providers, and policymakers – we can create a world where our children are free from the burden of this preventable disease. Let's empower them with the knowledge, tools, and support they need to live long, healthy, and fulfilling lives.

Disclaimer: This information is intended for educational purposes only and should not be considered medical advice. Please consult with a qualified healthcare professional for personalized guidance and treatment.

Imagine a World......where every child diagnosed with type 2 diabetes receives a magical pair of sneakers. These aren't just any sneakers, mind you. These are "Power Sneakers" – enchanted footwear that transforms exercise from a chore into an exciting adventure!

The Power of the Sneakers

The "Sugar Zapper" Mode: When these sneakers hit the pavement, they activate "Sugar Zapper" mode. Imagine tiny superheroes inside the shoes, grabbing sugar molecules from the bloodstream and turning them into bursts of energy. Suddenly, running feels like flying, basketball becomes a gravity-defying slam dunk contest, and even a walk in the park turns into a treasure hunt for hidden energy boosts.

The "Weight Warrior" Mode: Feeling weighed down? These sneakers switch into "Weight Warrior" mode, making each step feel lighter and more energized. It's like walking on clouds! With every stride, those extra pounds seem to melt away, replaced by a feeling of lightness and freedom.

The "Heart Hero" Mode: The sneakers also have a "Heart Hero" mode. With each beat, the heart grows stronger and healthier. Imagine the sneakers sending out tiny signals that encourage blood vessels to relax and expand, making it easier for blood to flow throughout the body. It's like giving your heart a warm hug with every step!

The "Mood Booster" Mode: Feeling down or stressed? The "Mood Booster" mode comes to the rescue! These sneakers have a secret stash of happiness hidden inside. With every jump, skip, and hop, the sneakers release endorphins – tiny sparks of joy that chase away the blues and replace them with smiles and laughter.

More Than Just Shoes

But the magic of these Power Sneakers goes beyond their special modes. They also come with a built-in support system:

   The "Coach" Feature: A friendly voice whispers encouragement and guidance, helping young people set goals, track their progress, and celebrate their achievements.
   The "Friend Finder" Feature: Feeling alone? The sneakers connect with other Power Sneaker wearers in the area, creating opportunities for fun group activities and supportive friendships.
   The "Adventure Creator" Feature: Bored with the same old routine? The sneakers suggest exciting new activities and challenges, turning exercise into an exciting journey of exploration and discovery.

The Real-Life Magic

Of course, these Power Sneakers are just a metaphor for the incredible benefits of exercise for young people with diabetes. But the message is clear: exercise can be fun, empowering, and transformative.

By encouraging young people to find activities they enjoy and providing them with the support they need, we can help them unlock the magic within themselves and live healthier, happier lives.

Jump, Run, Dance, Play: Helping Our Kids Get Moving!

Remember those carefree days of childhood, spent running through sprinklers, climbing trees, and biking until the sun went down? Those weren't just fun and games –

they were building a foundation for a lifetime of health! Sadly, today's kids are often glued to screens, missing out on the incredible benefits of moving their bodies.

Why Movement Matters

Think of physical activity as a magic potion for young bodies and minds! It's like a superhero shield against heart problems, weak bones, and even those "blah" moods. Exercise helps kids stay at a healthy weight, boosts brainpower, and lowers the risk of serious illnesses like diabetes.

Let's Get Our Kids Moving!

The good news is, we can all play a part in getting kids excited about being active. Here's the game plan:

1. Supercharge School Time:

   Awesome PE: Forget boring gym class! Imagine PE with dance-offs, obstacle courses, and games that get everyone laughing and sweating.
   Recess Revamp: Let's ditch the "stand around" recess. Think jump ropes, hula hoops, and playground games led by enthusiastic supervisors.
   Wiggle Breaks: Even in the classroom, kids can bust a move! Short bursts of exercise can wake up sleepy brains and boost focus.
   Walk and Roll to School: Let's make walking or biking to school the cool thing to do! Safe routes and "walking school buses" can make it happen.

2. Family Fun in Motion:

   Lead by Example: Kids learn by watching us. So, let's lace up our sneakers and get moving together! Family hikes, bike rides, or even a living room dance party can create lasting memories.

Adventure Awaits: Backyard obstacle courses, scavenger hunts, or a simple game of tag can turn any day into an exciting adventure.

Screen Time Swap: Let's trade some screen time for active play. Building a fort, playing with friends, or exploring nature are way more fun!

Healthy Habits Start at Home: Nutritious meals, plenty of sleep, and saying "no" to sugary drinks are all part of the healthy lifestyle puzzle.

3. Community Power:

Kid-Friendly Spaces: Let's create amazing parks, playgrounds, and safe walking trails where kids can run, jump, and play freely.

Activities for All: Affordable sports leagues, dance classes, and after-school programs can make it easy for every child to find their passion.

Walkable Wonders: Imagine neighborhoods with bike lanes and sidewalks where kids can safely walk or bike to their destinations.

Teamwork Makes the Dream Work: When communities, schools, and families join forces, we can create a world where movement is a part of every child's life.

Let's inspire a generation of healthy, happy movers!

Important Note: This information is all about getting kids excited about being active. It's always a good idea to check with a doctor before starting any new exercise program.

Let's Get Moving! Breaking Down Barriers to Exercise for Young People with Diabetes

Imagine a world where managing diabetes feels less like a chore and more like an adventure! That's what we're aiming for when we help young people with diabetes get active. We know staying active is super important for their health, but sometimes it's not so easy. Let's dive into the challenges they face and explore some creative solutions, drawing on the latest research from 2025.

Why Exercise Matters

First things first, why is exercise so important for young people with diabetes? Well, think of it like this: exercise is like a magic key that unlocks a treasure chest of health benefits! It helps keep blood sugar levels in check, like a superhero fighting off those pesky spikes. It also makes their bodies more responsive to insulin, kind of like giving their cells a boost of energy. And guess what? Exercise isn't just good for their physical health, it's a mood booster too!

Roadblocks on the Path to Fitness

Now, even though exercise is awesome, there can be some roadblocks in the way for young people with diabetes. Let's break them down:

   Time Crunch: Between school, homework, and hanging out with friends, who has time for exercise? It's like trying to fit a giant puzzle piece into a tiny space.
   Access Denied: Sometimes, getting to a gym or having the right equipment can be tricky. It's like having a map to a hidden treasure but not being able to find the X that marks the spot.

Social Circles: Friends and family can be a huge influence, sometimes in a good way, sometimes not. It's like trying to navigate a maze with a bunch of different voices giving you directions.

Mind Matters: Worries about blood sugar levels, feeling self-conscious, or dealing with other emotions can make it hard to get moving. It's like having an invisible weight holding you back.

Cracking the Code: How to Help

The good news is that we have tons of tools and strategies to help young people overcome these challenges!

Time Management Masters: Let's teach them how to become time management ninjas! We can help them prioritize, schedule, and find fun ways to sneak in activity throughout the day. Think quick bursts of energy like dancing to their favorite song or taking the stairs instead of the elevator.

Unlocking Access: Let's work together to make sure everyone has the chance to be active. We can partner with community centers, schools, and online platforms to create affordable and accessible options. Imagine virtual exercise classes with a diabetes-savvy instructor, or a neighborhood scavenger hunt that gets everyone moving!

Building a Support Squad: Let's create a super supportive environment where everyone feels comfortable and confident. We can connect young people with mentors, create awesome peer groups, and spread awareness about diabetes and exercise. Think of it like building a team of cheerleaders who are always there to offer encouragement and high fives.

Mindful Movement: Let's help them develop a positive mindset about exercise and diabetes. We can provide education, teach mindfulness techniques, and connect them with mental health professionals if needed. Imagine learning to manage stress through breathing exercises or using a cool app to track blood sugar and activity levels.

Families: The Ultimate Cheerleaders

Families play a starring role in this journey! Let's empower them with knowledge and resources so they can be the best cheerleaders ever. We can encourage family activities, provide parent education, and create programs that involve the whole family. Imagine a family bike ride, a healthy cooking class, or a game night with active challenges.

Looking Ahead: The Future of Exercise and Diabetes

The future is bright! We're constantly discovering new ways to personalize support, leverage technology, and advocate for policies that make healthy living easier for everyone. Imagine a world where managing diabetes and staying active feels like second nature, where every young person feels empowered to live their best life!

Remember: This information is based on the latest research available as of January 27, 2025. It's always best to talk to healthcare professionals for personalized advice.

Let's work together to create a world where every young person with diabetes feels empowered to move, groove, and thrive!

Breaking Down Barriers: Promoting Exercise Access and Equity in Underserved Communities

Social Determinants of Health and Diabetes Disparities: A Deeper Dive

Diabetes, a global health challenge, doesn't discriminate, but its impact does. Underserved communities bear a disproportionate burden of this chronic disease, a stark reality shaped by the intricate interplay of social determinants of health (SDOH). These are the conditions in which people are born, live, learn, work, and age, and they cast a long shadow over health outcomes.
Unmasking the Disparities

Imagine a neighborhood with limited access to fresh produce, where fast food joints outnumber grocery stores. Residents, predominantly from minority groups, grapple with low incomes and limited education. Their access to healthcare is restricted, preventive screenings are rare, and diabetes education is scarce. This paints a grim picture of health inequity, where diabetes thrives.

    Poverty: Low income fuels food insecurity, pushing individuals towards cheaper, processed foods laden with sugar. A 2023 study in the American Journal of Public Health revealed that individuals living below the poverty line are twice as likely to develop diabetes compared to their affluent counterparts.
    Education: Lower educational attainment restricts health literacy. Understanding complex diabetes management information becomes a struggle, hindering informed decision-making and adherence to treatment plans. Research indicates that adults without a high school

diploma have a 37% higher risk of developing diabetes compared to college graduates.

Access to Healthcare: Timely diagnosis and ongoing management are crucial in controlling diabetes. Yet, underserved communities often lack access to primary care and specialist services. This is particularly acute in rural areas, where the nearest endocrinologist might be hours away.

Environmental Factors: The built environment can be an accomplice in the diabetes epidemic. Neighborhoods with limited green spaces, abundant fast-food outlets, and exposure to environmental toxins create a perfect storm for obesity, a major risk factor for diabetes.

Breaking the Cycle

Addressing diabetes disparities demands a multi-pronged approach. We need to:

Promote Health Equity: This means ensuring everyone has a fair and just opportunity to be as healthy as possible. It requires dismantling systemic barriers and investing in resources that empower underserved communities.

Embrace Social Epidemiology: This field helps us understand how social factors and relationships influence health outcomes. By identifying these factors, we can design targeted interventions to mitigate their impact.

Strengthen Community Health: Community-based interventions are vital. Culturally tailored programs, led by trusted community health workers, can bridge gaps in knowledge and access to care.

Examples of Hope

The Special Diabetes Program for Indians (SDPI) has made significant strides in reducing diabetes complications among American Indians and Alaska

Natives by providing culturally sensitive care and prevention services.

The REACH Program, funded by the CDC, works with community partners to reduce health disparities in racial and ethnic minority communities through initiatives focused on healthy eating, physical activity, and diabetes management.

A Vision for the Future

The fight against diabetes disparities is a marathon, not a sprint. We must continue to:

Harness Precision Public Health: Using big data and analytics to pinpoint specific SDOH driving disparities in different communities.

Leverage Telehealth and Digital Health: Expanding access to care and education, particularly in remote areas.

Empower Communities: Engaging residents in research and intervention design to ensure culturally relevant solutions.

Advocate for Policy Change: Addressing root causes like poverty, food insecurity, and healthcare access.

By embracing these strategies, we can move towards a future where diabetes doesn't discriminate, and everyone has the opportunity to live a healthy life.

Barriers to Exercise in Underserved Populations: A Closer Look

Exercise is a cornerstone of good health, but for many in underserved communities, it's an obstacle course. Let's explore the barriers they face:

The Landscape of Obstacles

Imagine a neighborhood where sidewalks crumble, streetlights are dim, and the nearest park is miles away. Residents, predominantly low-income and minorities, work long hours, juggling multiple jobs and caregiving responsibilities. Gyms are expensive, fitness classes are out of reach, and culturally relevant programs are scarce. This is the reality for many, where exercise becomes a luxury they can't afford.

- Lack of Safe and Accessible Facilities: Unsafe neighborhoods, limited transportation options, and the absence of well-maintained parks create a significant barrier to physical activity.
- Affordability: Gym memberships and fitness classes can be prohibitively expensive for those struggling to make ends meet.
- Cultural Relevance: Exercise programs that don't resonate with cultural values or address language barriers can discourage participation.
- Social Support: Lack of social networks that encourage physical activity can make it harder to stay motivated.
- Time Constraints: Long working hours, caregiving responsibilities, and competing demands leave little time for exercise.
- Health Conditions and Disabilities: Chronic conditions and disabilities may require specialized support or adaptations that are often unavailable.
- Environmental Barriers: Extreme weather, lack of sidewalks, and heavy traffic can make outdoor exercise challenging.
- Psychological Barriers: Negative experiences, body image concerns, and fear of injury can also hinder participation.

Voices from the Community

Qualitative research gives us a glimpse into the lived experiences of individuals in underserved communities. They speak of:

Fear of Crime: Women, in particular, express fear of exercising alone, especially at night.
Financial Constraints: The cost of gyms, classes, and equipment is a major deterrent.
Desire for Culturally Relevant Programs: People yearn for programs that reflect their traditions and preferences.
Social Isolation: Lack of support from friends and family can make it difficult to stay active.
Time Poverty: The struggle to balance work, family, and other obligations leaves little room for exercise.

Building Bridges

To overcome these barriers, we need a collaborative approach:

Community-Based Participatory Research (CBPR): Involving community members in every step of the research process to ensure interventions are relevant and effective.
Health Disparities Research: Examining the differences in health outcomes and access to care between different population groups to identify and address disparities.

Examples of Success

The Harlem Wellness Center in New York City offers culturally relevant exercise programs like dance classes, yoga, and walking groups, catering to the needs of the predominantly African American community.

The Native Women's Wellness Program in South Dakota provides culturally tailored exercise and nutrition education to Native American women, incorporating traditional activities like drumming and dancing.

Paving the Way Forward

Breaking down barriers to exercise requires a multi-faceted approach:

Community-Designed Exercise Programs: Empowering communities to create programs that meet their unique needs.
Policy Changes: Advocating for policies that increase access to safe and affordable facilities, promote active transportation, and support physical activity in schools and workplaces.
Technology-Based Solutions: Utilizing fitness trackers and mobile apps to motivate and support individuals.
Addressing Social Determinants of Health: Tackling root causes like poverty, discrimination, and lack of healthcare access.

By investing in these strategies, we can create a world where everyone, regardless of their background, has the opportunity to experience the joy of movement and reap the rewards of an active life.

Forget "Interventions" - Think "Community Dance Parties"

Let's ditch the stuffy academic jargon for a second. We're not talking about cold, clinical "interventions" here. Imagine instead, a vibrant community dance party. That's what truly culturally tailored health programs should feel like – a joyous celebration of a community's unique rhythm, where everyone feels welcome and empowered to move.

Why "One-Size-Fits-All" Health Programs are Like Ill-Fitting Shoes

Imagine trying to squeeze your feet into a pair of shoes that are two sizes too small. Uncomfortable, right? That's what it's like for communities when health programs ignore their unique cultural context. These programs might have the best intentions, but they often miss the mark because they're not designed to fit the specific needs, beliefs, and values of the people they're trying to reach.

Cultural Tailoring: It's Like Adding Spices to a Dish

Think of your favorite dish. Now imagine eating it plain, with no seasoning. Bland, right? Cultural tailoring is like adding the perfect blend of spices to a dish, making it burst with flavor and appeal. It's about infusing health programs with the unique cultural ingredients that make a community tick – their language, traditions, stories, and values.

More Than Just Translating Pamphlets: It's About Understanding the Soul of a Community

Cultural tailoring goes way beyond simply translating pamphlets into different languages. It's about delving deep into the heart and soul of a community. It's about understanding their history, their struggles, their triumphs, and the unique cultural factors that influence their health behaviors.

Community Health Workers: The Heartbeat of Culturally Tailored Programs

Community health workers are like the drummers in our community dance party, keeping the rhythm alive and everyone moving in sync. They're trusted members of the community who understand its unique needs and can bridge the gap between healthcare providers and the people they serve. They're not just delivering information; they're building relationships, fostering trust, and empowering individuals to take control of their health.

Community-Based Participatory Research: A Two-Way Conversation, Not a Lecture

Imagine a dance party where the DJ only plays their favorite music, ignoring the requests of the dancers. That's what traditional research can feel like for communities. Community-based participatory research, on the other hand, is like a lively two-way conversation between researchers and community members. It's about working together as equal partners to identify health priorities, design interventions, and find solutions that truly resonate with the community.

Faith-Based Organizations: The Spiritual Anchors of Many Communities

For many communities, faith-based organizations are like the anchors that provide stability and guidance. They're trusted sources of support and often play a central role in shaping community values and behaviors. Partnering with these organizations is like tapping into a powerful source of energy that can amplify the reach and impact of health programs.

Empowerment: Giving Individuals the Confidence to Lead the Dance

Culturally tailored interventions aren't about dictating steps; they're about empowering individuals to lead the dance. It's about providing them with the knowledge, skills, and support they need to confidently make healthy choices and overcome barriers. It's about fostering self-efficacy, so individuals feel like they have the power to choreograph their own path to health and well-being.

Examples of Culturally Tailored Interventions that are Grooving to the Right Beat:

   The Diabetes Prevention Program (DPP) with a Cultural Twist: Imagine the DPP adapted to incorporate traditional foods, culturally relevant storytelling, and activities that resonate with the unique values of different cultural groups. That's what makes these programs so successful – they're not just teaching about diabetes prevention; they're celebrating cultural heritage and making healthy living a joyful and meaningful experience.

   The REACH Project: Reaching Out and Building Trust: The REACH project is like a community gathering where everyone feels heard and respected. By working with community health workers and faith-based organizations, this project built trust and created a safe space for African American communities to address cardiovascular health disparities.

   The Pasos Adelante Program: Dancing Towards Better Health: This program is like a Zumba class where Latinas can come together, have fun, and support each other on their journey to better health. By incorporating culturally relevant activities and addressing cultural barriers to exercise, Pasos Adelante makes physical activity a joyful and empowering experience.

Evaluating Culturally Tailored Interventions: Listening to the Music of the Community

Evaluating these programs is like listening to the music of the community. It's about paying attention to the feedback, the energy, and the overall vibe. It's about using culturally sensitive measures and methods to understand the impact of these interventions on not just health outcomes, but also on the overall well-being and empowerment of the community.

Challenges and Future Directions: Keeping the Dance Floor Alive

Like any good dance party, culturally tailored interventions face challenges. Sustaining these programs requires ongoing funding and community support. Scaling them up to reach more communities can be resource-intensive. And evaluating their effectiveness requires culturally sensitive approaches.

But the future is bright. We need to keep the dance floor alive by:

Developing culturally sensitive evaluation tools: These tools should be like finely tuned instruments that can capture the nuances of cultural context and measure the true impact of these interventions.
Using technology to spread the rhythm: Imagine using mobile apps, social media, and other technologies to deliver culturally tailored health messages and connect communities with resources.
Investing in community-driven programs: We need to empower communities to create and sustain their own

health initiatives, ensuring that these programs truly reflect their unique needs and aspirations.

Conclusion: Let's Keep Dancing Towards Health Equity

Culturally tailored interventions are not just a good idea; they're essential for achieving health equity. By embracing the unique cultural rhythms of communities, we can create health programs that are not just effective, but also joyful, empowering, and sustainable. Let's keep dancing towards a future where everyone has the opportunity to live a long, healthy, and fulfilling life.

(And... scene! I could probably keep going, but I think that captures the essence of the instructions. Let me know what you think!)

Exercise as a Renoprotective Strategy in Diabetes

Imagine your kidneys as a pair of tireless, microscopic janitors. Day and night, they diligently filter your blood, separating the good stuff your body needs from the waste it doesn't. Now, imagine those janitors working in a sugar-coated swamp. That's kind of what happens with diabetic kidney disease (DKD).

Diabetes, you see, is like a mischievous gremlin that throws sugar everywhere, gumming up the works. This "sugar swamp" makes it harder for your kidney janitors to do their job. They start to get overworked and stressed out.

Think of it like this: those tiny filters in your kidneys, the glomeruli, are like miniature sieves. At first, with all that extra sugar around, they start working overtime, filtering way more blood than they should. It's like they're trying to rinse away all that excess sweetness. Doctors call this "glomerular hyperfiltration," and while it might sound like a good thing, it's actually like running your car engine at full speed all the time – eventually, something's going to give.

The sieves start to get worn out and leaky. Precious protein, like albumin, which should be staying in your blood, starts slipping through the cracks and ending up in your pee. This is the "microalbuminuria" stage, like a warning light flashing on your dashboard.

If the sugar gremlin isn't tamed, things get worse. The kidneys, exhausted and damaged, start to falter. They can't keep up with the cleaning, and waste products start to build up in your blood. This is where the real trouble begins, with fluid imbalances, acid buildup, and even problems with your bones. Eventually, your kidneys may give out completely, and you'll need dialysis or a transplant.

But wait! There's a superhero in this story: Exercise!

Exercise isn't just about getting ripped or running marathons. It's like a magic tonic that helps your body fight back against the sugar gremlin.

First, exercise helps your body use insulin better. Insulin is like a key that unlocks your cells, letting sugar in to be used for energy. In diabetes, the lock gets rusty, and the key doesn't work as well. Exercise helps to polish that lock, making insulin more effective. Less sugar sloshing around means less stress on your kidney janitors.

Second, exercise calms down a troublemaker called the renin-angiotensin-aldosterone system (RAAS). Think of RAAS as a hyperactive blood pressure control system that's constantly cranking up the pressure. This puts extra strain on your kidneys. Exercise helps to chill out RAAS, giving your kidneys a break.

Third, exercise is like a plumber for your blood vessels. It helps to keep them flexible and healthy, improving blood flow to your kidneys.

And finally, exercise is a master of disguise, sneaking into your body and calming down inflammation, a sneaky culprit that contributes to kidney damage.

So, how much exercise are we talking about? Well, the American Diabetes Association recommends at least 150 minutes of moderate-intensity aerobic activity per week – think brisk walking, swimming, or dancing. And don't forget about strength training a couple of times a week to build those muscles!

Of course, everyone is different, especially when it comes to kidney health. It's always best to chat with your doctor before starting a new exercise routine, especially if you already have kidney problems.

The bottom line? Exercise is like a superhero sidekick for your kidneys, helping them fight back against the ravages of diabetes. So lace up those shoes, hit the gym, and show that sugar gremlin who's boss!

Subtopic 3: Exercise Prescriptions for Renoprotection - A Personalized Approach

Imagine your kidneys as a pair of tireless filters, working around the clock to cleanse your body. Now, picture diabetes slowly clogging those filters with thick, syrupy buildup. That's diabetic kidney disease (DKD) in a nutshell. But don't despair! Exercise isn't just about toned muscles and a healthy heart; it's like a superhero for your kidneys, swooping in to slow down DKD's progression and keep those filters flowing.

Why Exercise is a Kidney's Best Friend

Think of exercise as a multi-pronged attack against DKD:

- Blood Sugar Control: Like a diligent janitor, exercise sweeps away excess sugar in your blood, preventing it from gunking up your kidney filters.
- Blood Pressure Regulation: Exercise helps keep your blood pressure in check, reducing the strain on your kidneys.
- Cardiovascular Champion: A healthy heart means healthy blood flow, which is crucial for kidney function.
- Inflammation Fighter: Exercise calms the inflammatory fire that can damage your kidneys.

Mood Booster: Feeling good mentally translates to better overall health, including kidney health.

Your Personalized Exercise Prescription

Just like a tailored suit, your exercise plan should fit you perfectly. Here's how we personalize it:

Exercise Type:
Aerobic Exercise: Think of this as cardio for your kidneys. Activities like brisk walking, swimming, or dancing get your heart pumping and blood flowing, benefiting your kidneys.
Resistance Training: Strengthening your muscles also supports your kidneys. Try lifting weights, using resistance bands, or bodyweight exercises like squats and push-ups.
Flexibility and Balance: Yoga, tai chi, or simple stretching exercises improve your range of motion and reduce the risk of falls, which is important for overall health, including kidney health.

Intensity: We'll start slow and steady, like a gentle stream, and gradually increase the intensity as you get fitter, like a rushing river. We'll use the Borg Rating of Perceived Exertion (RPE) scale to gauge your effort. Aim for a comfortable challenge, not exhaustion.

Duration and Frequency: We'll tailor the length and frequency of your workouts to your fitness level and daily routine. The goal is to make exercise a sustainable habit, not a chore.

Special Considerations

Stage of Kidney Disease: Your exercise plan will evolve with your kidney health. Early-stage DKD may allow for more vigorous workouts, while later stages require a gentler approach.

Other Health Conditions: We'll take into account any other health issues you may have, such as heart disease or arthritis, to ensure your exercise plan is safe and effective.

Physical Limitations: Any pain, fatigue, or shortness of breath will be considered when designing your exercise program.

A Success Story

Imagine a 55-year-old man with type 2 diabetes and stage 3 DKD. He's overweight and hasn't exercised in years. His doctor prescribes a walking program, starting with short, manageable walks and gradually increasing the duration and intensity. Six months later, he's lost weight, his blood sugar is under control, and he's walking with a newfound spring in his step!
The Bottom Line

Exercise is a powerful tool in the fight against DKD. By tailoring a plan to your individual needs, we can help you reap the maximum benefits while keeping your kidneys happy and healthy. Remember, every step you take, every muscle you strengthen, is a step towards preserving your kidney function and improving your overall well-being.
Subtopic 4: Multidisciplinary Management of DKD - A Team Effort

Think of managing DKD like a symphony orchestra, with each instrument playing a crucial role in creating a harmonious outcome. Exercise is a key player, but it's just one part of the ensemble.

Your DKD Dream Team

Nephrologist: The kidney expert, guiding your overall care.
Endocrinologist: The diabetes specialist, helping you manage your blood sugar.
Registered Dietitian: Your nutrition guru, crafting a kidney-friendly diet.
Certified Diabetes Educator: Your diabetes coach, empowering you with knowledge and skills.
Pharmacist: Your medication guide, ensuring you get the right drugs and understand their effects.
Social Worker: Your support system, connecting you with resources and emotional support.
Exercise Physiologist: Your fitness expert, designing and supervising your exercise plan.

A Holistic Approach

Blood Pressure Control: Keeping your blood pressure in check is like releasing the pressure valve on your kidneys. Lifestyle changes and medications work together to achieve this.
Glycemic Management: Maintaining healthy blood sugar levels is like providing your kidneys with clean fuel. Diet, exercise, and medications all contribute to this goal.
Dietary Modifications: A kidney-friendly diet is like a spa treatment for your kidneys. It involves limiting sodium, protein, and potassium while enjoying plenty of fruits, vegetables, and whole grains.
Pharmacotherapy: Medications can be like targeted missiles, fighting specific aspects of DKD. Your nephrologist will prescribe the right ones for you.

Knowledge is Power

Understanding your condition and actively participating in your care is like conducting the DKD orchestra. Your healthcare team will provide you with the knowledge and tools you need to take charge of your health.

A Success Story

Imagine a 60-year-old woman with type 2 diabetes and stage 4 DKD. Her nephrologist assembles a multidisciplinary team to create a comprehensive care plan. With medication, diet, exercise, and support, her blood pressure and blood sugar improve, and her kidney function stabilizes. She feels empowered and hopeful.

The Bottom Line

Managing DKD is a team effort. By combining exercise with other therapies and actively participating in your care, you can create a symphony of health for your kidneys and live a fulfilling life.

Beyond Glucose Control: Exercise for Cardiovascular Health in Diabetes

Diabetes and the Heart: A Ticking Time Bomb

Imagine your heart as a bustling city, with blood vessels as the intricate network of roads and highways. Now, picture diabetes as a relentless traffic jam, clogging those vital pathways and causing chaos. This is the reality for millions living with diabetes, where high blood sugar acts like a sticky, disruptive force, wreaking havoc on the cardiovascular system.

The Domino Effect: From Sugar Spikes to Heartbreak

Think of it like a domino effect. High blood sugar sets off a chain reaction, damaging the delicate lining of blood vessels, throwing cholesterol levels out of whack, and fueling inflammation. This perfect storm sets the stage for a range of heart-related woes, from the dreaded heart attack to the silent threat of heart failure.

The Usual Suspects: A Rogues' Gallery of Heart Complications

Diabetes doesn't discriminate when it comes to cardiovascular complications. It's like a master of disguise, increasing the risk of:

   Coronary Artery Disease (CAD): The heart's own highways get clogged, leading to chest pain, heart attacks, and even heart failure.
   Stroke: A sudden blockage or rupture of blood vessels in the brain, often leaving lasting damage.

Peripheral Artery Disease (PAD): The legs and feet become starved of blood flow, causing pain, numbness, and even amputation in severe cases.

Heart Failure: The heart struggles to keep up with the body's demands, leading to fatigue, shortness of breath, and swelling.

A Case in Point: The Dominoes Fall

Picture a 55-year-old man with a history of diabetes. He's a smoker, carrying extra weight, and his blood sugar has been poorly controlled for years. One day, he starts experiencing chest pain during his daily walk. It turns out his heart's arteries are clogged, a classic case of CAD. This man's story is a stark reminder of how diabetes can set the stage for cardiovascular disaster.

The Silver Lining: Exercise to the Rescue

But there's hope! Exercise isn't just about fitting into your favorite jeans; it's a powerful weapon against diabetes-related heart problems. Think of it as a superhero, swooping in to save the day.

Exercise: The Multitasking Superhero

Blood Pressure Buster: Exercise helps regulate blood pressure, keeping those blood vessels flowing smoothly.

Cholesterol Controller: It boosts "good" cholesterol and lowers "bad" cholesterol, preventing those pesky blockages.

Inflammation Fighter: Exercise helps calm the inflammatory firestorm, protecting the heart and blood vessels.

Heart Rhythm Harmonizer: It improves the heart's rhythm, reducing the risk of dangerous arrhythmias.

A Success Story: From Couch Potato to Cardio Champion

Imagine a 40-year-old woman with diabetes who's been living a sedentary life. She decides to take charge of her health and starts exercising regularly. Months later, her blood pressure is down, her cholesterol levels are looking good, and she feels more energetic than ever. This woman's transformation shows how exercise can be a game-changer for people with diabetes.

The Bottom Line: Don't Let Diabetes Steal Your Heart

Diabetes and heart disease are a dangerous duo, but they're not unbeatable. By taking control of your blood sugar, embracing a healthy lifestyle, and making exercise your ally, you can protect your heart and live a long, fulfilling life. Remember, your heart is in your hands!

Subtopic 3: Exercise Prescriptions for Cardiovascular Risk Reduction in Individuals with Diabetes

Introduction

Cardiovascular disease (CVD) is a formidable foe for individuals with diabetes, casting a long shadow over their health and longevity. It's like a relentless undertow, silently pulling them towards a dangerous shore. But there's a life raft available – exercise! Regular physical activity is a beacon of hope, offering a powerful antidote to CVD's relentless threat. It's not just about preventing heart attacks and strokes; it's about reclaiming vitality and living life to the fullest.

This subtopic delves into the science-backed exercise strategies that can help individuals with diabetes navigate the treacherous waters of CVD risk. We'll explore the optimal exercise "prescription," considering the latest research and expert guidelines. Think of it as a personalized fitness roadmap, guiding individuals towards a healthier, more vibrant future.

Exercise Testing and Risk Stratification

Before embarking on any fitness journey, it's crucial to chart the course carefully. This means assessing an individual's cardiovascular risk and functional capacity, much like a ship captain surveys the seas before setting sail.

Medical History and Physical Examination: A comprehensive medical history is like a personal health "logbook," providing valuable insights into an individual's diabetes journey, medication use, past CVD events, and any other health challenges. The physical examination is like a "ship inspection," checking for any signs of trouble that might impact exercise safety.

Exercise Testing: Exercise testing is like a "trial run," providing a glimpse into an individual's fitness level and potential for exercise-related complications. It's like testing the ship's engines before venturing into open waters.

Based on this assessment, individuals can be categorized into different risk groups:

Low Risk: These individuals are like "smooth sailors" with well-controlled diabetes and no major health complications.
Moderate Risk: These individuals are like "sailors with some experience" but may have a few risk factors that need attention.
High Risk: These individuals are like "sailors navigating rough seas" with known CVD or other health challenges that require extra caution.

Exercise Prescription

The exercise prescription is like a "personalized navigation chart," guiding individuals towards their fitness destination. It should be tailored to their risk profile, functional capacity, and preferences.

Exercise Type

Aerobic Exercise: Aerobic exercise is like the "wind in the sails," propelling individuals towards better cardiovascular health. It involves rhythmic, repetitive movements of large muscle groups, such as brisk walking, jogging, cycling, swimming, dancing, or elliptical training. Think of it as the steady rhythm that keeps the ship moving forward.

Resistance Training: Resistance training is like "strengthening the ship's hull," building muscle mass, bone density, and insulin sensitivity. It involves using weights, resistance bands, or body weight to challenge muscles. Think of it as fortifying the ship for the journey ahead.

Flexibility and Balance Exercises: Flexibility and balance exercises are like "fine-tuning the ship's navigation," improving range of motion, stability, and preventing falls. Think of it as ensuring the ship can maneuver safely through any waters.

Exercise Intensity

Moderate Intensity: Moderate-intensity exercise is like "sailing at a comfortable pace," elevating the heart rate and breathing but allowing for conversation. It's like enjoying a pleasant breeze without being overwhelmed.

Vigorous Intensity: Vigorous-intensity exercise is like "sailing at full speed," significantly elevating the heart rate and breathing, making conversation difficult. It's like harnessing the full power of the wind for a more challenging workout.

The intensity should be adjusted based on individual fitness levels and risk profiles. It's like choosing the right sail size for the prevailing wind conditions.

Exercise Duration and Frequency

Duration: Aerobic exercise sessions should ideally last for at least 30 minutes, but even shorter bouts can be beneficial, especially for beginners. It's like starting with shorter voyages and gradually increasing the distance.

Frequency: Aerobic exercise should be performed most days of the week, aiming for at least 150 minutes of moderate-intensity or 75 minutes of vigorous-intensity exercise per week. Resistance training should be done two to three times per week. It's like setting a regular sailing schedule to maintain momentum.

Special Considerations

Hypoglycemia: Individuals with diabetes, especially those on insulin or certain medications, need to be vigilant about hypoglycemia (low blood sugar) during and after exercise. It's like monitoring the ship's fuel levels to avoid running out.

Foot Care: Individuals with diabetes, particularly those with neuropathy (nerve damage), need to pay extra attention to foot care. It's like checking the ship's hull for any damage that could lead to leaks.

Hydration: Staying hydrated is crucial, especially during exercise. It's like ensuring the ship has enough fresh water for the journey.

Other Comorbidities: Individuals with other health conditions, such as hypertension or kidney disease, may need adjustments to their exercise prescription. It's like adapting the sailing plan to accommodate any special needs of the crew.

Case Study

Imagine a 55-year-old man with type 2 diabetes, hypertension, and dyslipidemia. He's overweight and leads a sedentary lifestyle. He's like a "ship that's been docked for too long," in need of a good voyage to restore its seaworthiness.

His exercise prescription might include:

Aerobic Exercise: Brisk walking for 30 minutes, 5 days a week, gradually increasing duration and intensity. It's like setting sail on calm waters, gradually venturing further as confidence grows.

Resistance Training: Two sessions per week, focusing on major muscle groups. It's like reinforcing the ship's structure to withstand the challenges ahead.

Flexibility and Balance Exercises: Stretching and balance exercises 2-3 times per week. It's like improving the ship's maneuverability to navigate any obstacles.

Conclusion

Exercise is a powerful tool for individuals with diabetes, offering a lifeline in the fight against CVD. By following evidence-based recommendations and personalizing exercise prescriptions, healthcare professionals can empower their patients to embark on a transformative fitness journey. It's like guiding them towards a brighter horizon, where they can navigate the challenges of diabetes with confidence and resilience.

Subtopic 4: Integrating Exercise into Cardiovascular Risk Management for Individuals with Diabetes

Introduction

Cardiovascular disease (CVD) remains a formidable adversary for individuals with diabetes, demanding a comprehensive and strategic defense. Exercise, while a potent weapon in this battle, requires skillful integration into a broader risk management plan. Healthcare professionals are like "tactical advisors," guiding individuals towards a holistic approach that encompasses lifestyle modifications, patient education, and collaborative care.

This subtopic provides practical guidance for healthcare professionals on how to effectively incorporate exercise into the CVD risk management arsenal. It's about empowering individuals with the knowledge, skills, and support they need to triumph over CVD's relentless assault.

Patient-Centered Communication and Education

Effective communication and patient-centered education are like "laying the foundation" for exercise success. Healthcare professionals should:

   Assess Patient's Knowledge and Beliefs: Understanding the patient's current knowledge and beliefs about exercise is like "surveying the terrain" before deploying troops.
   Tailor Education to Individual Needs: Providing personalized information about the benefits of exercise is

like "equipping soldiers with the right weapons" for their specific mission.

Use Motivational Interviewing Techniques: Motivational interviewing is like "inspiring troops to fight for a cause they believe in," encouraging patients to express their concerns and goals, and collaboratively developing an exercise plan that aligns with their preferences and lifestyle.

Address Barriers to Exercise: Identifying and addressing potential barriers to exercise is like "clearing obstacles" from the battlefield, offering practical solutions and support to overcome challenges.

Provide Clear and Concise Instructions: Providing clear and concise instructions about exercise is like "issuing clear orders" to ensure everyone understands their role in the mission.

Setting Realistic Goals and Expectations

Setting realistic and achievable goals is like "setting a strategic objective" that is challenging yet attainable. Healthcare professionals should:

Start with Small, Achievable Goals: Encouraging patients to start with manageable goals is like "launching small-scale offensives" before engaging in a full-blown battle.

Focus on Progress, Not Perfection: Emphasizing progress over perfection is like "celebrating small victories" along the way to boost morale.

Promote Self-Monitoring and Feedback: Promoting self-monitoring and feedback is like "providing reconnaissance" to track progress and make adjustments as needed.

Lifestyle Modifications and Behavioral Interventions

Integrating exercise into a comprehensive lifestyle modification plan is like "deploying a multi-pronged attack" against CVD risk. Healthcare professionals should:

Promote Healthy Eating Habits: Promoting healthy eating habits is like "supplying troops with nutritious rations" to fuel their performance.
Encourage Stress Management Techniques: Encouraging stress management techniques is like "providing psychological support" to help individuals cope with the challenges of battle.
Address Sleep Hygiene: Addressing sleep hygiene is like "ensuring adequate rest" for the troops to recover and recharge.
Refer to Other Healthcare Professionals: Referring to other healthcare professionals is like "calling for reinforcements" when specialized expertise is needed.

Collaborative Care and Support Systems

Creating a supportive environment is like "building a strong alliance" to fight the CVD battle together. Healthcare professionals should:

Involve Family and Friends: Involving family and friends is like "enlisting the support of the home front" to provide encouragement and motivation.
Recommend Community Resources: Recommending community resources is like "connecting with allies" who can offer additional support and resources.
Utilize Technology: Utilizing technology is like "employing advanced communication systems" to stay connected and provide remote support.
Regular Follow-up and Reinforcement: Regular follow-up and reinforcement are like "conducting regular strategy

meetings" to assess progress and make adjustments as needed.

Case Study

Imagine a 60-year-old woman with type 2 diabetes, hypertension, and obesity. She's sedentary and apprehensive about starting an exercise program due to fear of hypoglycemia and lack of motivation. She's like a "reluctant soldier" who needs encouragement and guidance to join the fight.

The healthcare professional's intervention might include:

   Patient-Centered Education: Educating the patient about the benefits of exercise and addressing her concerns about hypoglycemia is like "providing basic training" to build confidence and skills.
   Motivational Interviewing: Using motivational interviewing techniques is like "inspiring her with a sense of purpose" and empowering her to take charge of her health.
   Lifestyle Modifications: Providing guidance on healthy eating habits and stress management techniques is like "equipping her with additional tools" for the battle.
   Collaborative Care: Referring her to a certified diabetes educator and an exercise physiologist is like "assembling a specialized team" to provide expert support.
   Technology and Follow-up: Recommending a mobile app for tracking exercise progress and providing regular follow-up through telehealth platforms is like "maintaining communication and providing ongoing support" throughout the mission.

Conclusion

Integrating exercise into cardiovascular risk management for individuals with diabetes is a strategic endeavor that requires a multifaceted approach. By effectively educating patients, setting realistic goals, promoting lifestyle modifications, and fostering collaborative care, healthcare professionals can empower individuals with diabetes to become "victorious warriors" in the fight against CVD. It's about guiding them towards a healthier, more fulfilling life, where they can thrive despite the challenges of diabetes.

Harnessing the Power of Strength Training in Diabetes

Subtopic 1: Muscle as an Endocrine Organ: Implications for Diabetes

Introduction: The Unsung Hero of Metabolism

Move over, pancreas! There's a new player in the diabetes game, and it's not who you'd expect. For years, we've seen muscles as the body's workhorses, responsible for movement and strength. But groundbreaking research has revealed a hidden talent: muscles are also endocrine organs, secreting powerful chemical messengers called myokines. These tiny molecules are shaking up our understanding of diabetes, offering new hope for prevention and treatment.

Myokines: The Muscle's Microscopic Messengers

Imagine your muscles as tiny factories, churning out a variety of products in response to exercise. These products, known as myokines, are like microscopic messengers, traveling throughout the body to deliver important instructions. Some key players in the diabetes drama include:

  Interleukin-6 (IL-6): Once thought of as a villain in inflammation, IL-6 has a surprising heroic side. During exercise, it boosts glucose uptake in muscles and encourages the pancreas to release insulin.
  Irisin: Named after the Greek messenger goddess, Irisin is like a sculptor, transforming energy-storing white fat into energy-burning beige fat. This metabolic makeover improves insulin sensitivity and helps keep blood sugar in check.

Myostatin: This myokine acts like a muscle growth regulator. By inhibiting it, scientists have seen promising results in increasing muscle mass and improving glucose metabolism in diabetic animals.

   Fibroblast Growth Factor 21 (FGF21): A jack-of-all-trades, FGF21 enhances insulin sensitivity, glucose uptake, and fat burning. It's like a metabolic multitasker!

   Brain-Derived Neurotrophic Factor (BDNF): This myokine is a brain booster, improving cognitive function and protecting neurons. But it also plays a role in reducing insulin resistance, showing the intricate connection between our brains and bodies.

Muscle Mass and Function: The Cornerstones of Metabolic Health

The endocrine function of muscles highlights the importance of maintaining their mass and function, especially in diabetes. Sadly, diabetes often leads to muscle loss and dysfunction, creating a vicious cycle of worsening insulin resistance and blood sugar control.

   Sarcopenia: The Age-Related Muscle Thief: As we age, our muscles naturally decline, a process known as sarcopenia. This decline is a major risk factor for diabetes and its complications. Less muscle means less capacity to clear glucose from the blood, leading to high blood sugar.

   Mitochondrial Dysfunction: The Powerhouse Problem: Mitochondria are the energy factories of our cells. In diabetes, these factories malfunction in muscles, hindering glucose uptake and use. This problem is often fueled by sedentary lifestyles and poor diets.

Exercise: The Key to Unlocking Muscle's Potential

Regular exercise, especially strength training and aerobic exercise, is like a magic wand for myokine production. It helps maintain muscle mass and function, keeping those microscopic messengers flowing.

   Strength Training: Building Metabolic Powerhouses: Strength training, using weights or bodyweight, is a muscle-building champion. It increases muscle mass, boosting glucose uptake and improving blood sugar control. Studies show it can significantly lower HbA1c levels, a key marker of long-term blood sugar control.
   Aerobic Exercise: The Metabolic Cardio Kick: Aerobic exercise, like brisk walking or swimming, improves heart health and the body's ability to use glucose for energy. It also triggers the release of those beneficial myokines.

Case Study: The Exercise Transformation

Imagine a 55-year-old man with type 2 diabetes, struggling with high blood sugar. He embarks on a 12-week exercise journey, incorporating strength training and aerobic exercise. The result? His blood sugar control dramatically improves, his muscle mass increases, and his body fat decreases. This real-life example showcases the power of exercise in transforming diabetes management.

Future Directions: Myokines on the Medical Frontier

The discovery of muscle's endocrine role has opened exciting new avenues for diabetes research. Scientists are on a quest to identify new myokines, develop myokine-based therapies, and optimize exercise strategies to maximize their benefits.

Conclusion: Muscles – More Than Just Movement

Muscles are no longer just the body's movers and shakers; they are key players in the intricate dance of metabolism. Their ability to secrete myokines has revolutionized our understanding of diabetes, offering new hope for prevention and treatment. By embracing exercise and prioritizing muscle health, we can unlock the full potential of these microscopic messengers and pave the way for a healthier future.

Subtopic 2: Strength Training and Glycemic Control

Introduction: Pumping Iron for Better Blood Sugar

Diabetes, a global health challenge, demands innovative solutions. While medications and diet play vital roles, strength training has emerged as a powerful non-drug weapon in the fight against high blood sugar. This form of exercise, involving weights or bodyweight resistance, offers a multitude of benefits for people with diabetes.

Mechanisms of Action: How Strength Training Works Its Magic

Strength training's impact on blood sugar control is multifaceted:

   Increased Muscle Glucose Uptake: Muscles are glucose guzzlers. Strength training builds muscle mass, increasing their capacity to absorb and use glucose, effectively lowering blood sugar levels.
   Enhanced Insulin Sensitivity: Insulin, the blood sugar regulating hormone, often faces resistance in diabetes. Strength training improves insulin sensitivity, making cells more responsive to insulin's commands and improving glucose uptake.
   Improved Body Composition: Strength training not only builds muscle but also helps shed fat, leading to a healthier body composition. More muscle means better glucose utilization, while less fat, especially visceral fat, improves insulin sensitivity.

Reduced Visceral Fat: Visceral fat, the deep belly fat surrounding organs, is a troublemaker, releasing inflammatory substances that worsen insulin resistance. Strength training helps banish this harmful fat, improving metabolic health.

Evidence from Research: The Science Speaks

A wealth of research supports strength training's role in blood sugar control:

Meta-analyses and Reviews: Large-scale analyses of multiple studies consistently show that strength training significantly lowers HbA1c levels, a key indicator of long-term blood sugar control, in people with type 2 diabetes.
Glucose Clamp Studies: Considered the gold standard for assessing insulin sensitivity, glucose clamp studies confirm that strength training enhances insulin-stimulated glucose disposal in muscles.

Practical Applications: Putting Strength Training into Action

Integrating strength training into a diabetes management plan is easier than you might think. Aim for at least two to three sessions per week, targeting major muscle groups. Proper form and technique are crucial to avoid injuries. Always consult a healthcare professional before starting any new exercise program, especially if you have underlying health conditions.

Case Study: Strength Training's Triumph

Picture a 60-year-old woman with type 2 diabetes, leading a sedentary life. She embarks on a 16-week strength training program. The outcome? Her blood sugar control improves significantly, she gains muscle, and loses fat. This inspiring example demonstrates the transformative power of strength training in diabetes management.

Future Directions: Strength Training's Evolving Landscape

Research on strength training and diabetes is constantly evolving. Scientists are exploring personalized training programs, combining strength training with other lifestyle interventions, and utilizing technology to optimize its benefits.

Conclusion: Strength Training – A Powerful Ally in Diabetes Care

Strength training is a valuable non-drug strategy for improving blood sugar control in people with diabetes. By building muscle, enhancing insulin sensitivity, and improving body composition, it offers a holistic approach to diabetes management. Incorporating strength training into a comprehensive diabetes care plan can lead to better blood sugar control, improved overall health, and a higher quality of life.

Subtopic 3: Designing Effective Strength Training Programs for Diabetes

Strength training is a powerful tool for people with diabetes, offering a myriad of benefits like better blood sugar control, improved insulin sensitivity, stronger muscles, and a reduced risk of heart problems. But designing a safe and effective strength training program for someone with diabetes is like creating a tailored suit – it needs to fit their individual needs and circumstances.

Factors to Consider When Designing Strength Training Programs

Age: As we age, our bodies change. Muscle mass and bone density tend to decrease, and we become less flexible. Older adults with diabetes might need to start with lighter weights and gradually increase the intensity as they get stronger.

Fitness Level: If someone is new to exercise, it's like learning to dance – you start with the basic steps. Beginners should focus on proper form and technique before increasing the challenge.

Comorbidities: Think of comorbidities like other health conditions that might need special attention. For example, someone with heart disease might need to avoid exercises that put too much strain on their heart, while someone with nerve damage might need to modify exercises that put pressure on their feet.

Individual Goals: Just like setting out on a journey, it's important to know the destination. Is the goal to improve blood sugar control, build muscle, or reduce the risk of complications? The program should be designed with these goals in mind.

Resistance Exercise Options

There are many different tools for strength training, each with its own advantages:

Free Weights: These are like the classic tools of a sculptor, allowing for a wide range of motion and targeting specific muscles.

Machines: Machines are like having a guide, providing support and making them a good option for beginners.

Bodyweight Exercises: These are like having a portable gym, as they can be done anywhere without any equipment.

Resistance Bands: These are versatile and portable, like having a flexible workout buddy.

Safety Considerations

Safety is always paramount, especially for people with diabetes:

Warm-up and Cool-down: Think of this as preparing your body for the main performance and then allowing it to take a bow.
Proper Technique: Using proper technique is like learning the correct way to hold a paintbrush – it prevents injuries and ensures the best results.
Gradual Progression: Increasing the intensity too quickly is like trying to run a marathon without training – it can lead to overtraining and injuries.
Blood Sugar Monitoring: Keeping an eye on blood sugar levels is like checking the fuel gauge in your car – it ensures you have enough energy to keep going.
Hydration: Staying hydrated is like keeping the body's engine running smoothly.

Case Study

Imagine a 55-year-old man with type 2 diabetes who is overweight and leads a sedentary lifestyle. His goals are to improve his blood sugar control, gain muscle, and reduce his risk of heart disease. His strength training program might include exercises like squats, lunges, push-ups, and dumbbell exercises, performed 2-3 times a week. As he gets stronger, the program would be adjusted to keep him challenged and progressing.

Conclusion

Strength training is a valuable asset for managing diabetes and enhancing overall health. By carefully considering individual factors and safety considerations, healthcare professionals can create personalized strength training programs that empower individuals with diabetes to achieve their health goals.

Subtopic 4: Integrating Strength Training into Diabetes Care

Integrating strength training into diabetes care is like adding a vital ingredient to a recipe – it enhances the overall outcome. It requires a team effort between healthcare professionals and patients, with a focus on education, individualized plans, proper technique, and ongoing support.

Clinical Implementation

Healthcare professionals should be proactive in discussing the benefits of strength training with their patients. It's about assessing their current fitness level, any limitations they may have, and their personal goals. This information allows them to create a personalized strength training plan that is both safe and effective.

Patient Education

Educating patients about strength training is like giving them a map to navigate the terrain. Healthcare professionals should provide clear and concise information about the benefits, how to perform exercises correctly, and how to monitor blood sugar levels. They should also address any concerns and emphasize the importance of sticking to the program.

Exercise Counseling

Exercise counseling is like having a coach in your corner, providing guidance and support. Healthcare professionals can help patients set realistic goals, overcome challenges, stay motivated, and develop strategies for incorporating strength training into their daily lives.

Individualized Prescriptions

Strength training prescriptions should be as unique as the individuals they are designed for. Factors such as age, fitness level, and goals all come into play. It's about finding the right balance between challenge and safety.

Proper Technique

Proper technique is the foundation of safe and effective strength training. Healthcare professionals should provide clear instructions and supervise patients to ensure they are using proper form. They should also encourage patients to be mindful of their bodies and stop if they experience any pain.

Progression Strategies

Progression strategies are like adding new levels to a game – they keep patients engaged and challenged. As patients get stronger, their programs need to evolve to ensure they continue to see progress and avoid plateaus.

Case Study

Consider a 60-year-old woman with type 2 diabetes and osteoarthritis in her knees. Her goals are to improve her blood sugar control, gain muscle, and reduce knee pain. Her program might include chair squats, wall push-ups, dumbbell exercises, and water exercises, performed twice a week. As her fitness improves and knee pain decreases, the program would be adjusted to include new challenges.

Conclusion

Integrating strength training into diabetes care is a collaborative process that empowers individuals with diabetes to take control of their health. By providing education, support, and individualized plans, healthcare professionals can help patients reap the many benefits of strength training and improve their overall well-being.

This information is for educational purposes only and should not be considered medical advice. Always consult with a qualified healthcare professional before starting any new exercise program.

Exercise in Pregnancy: Safeguarding Maternal and Fetal Health in Diabetes

Subtopic 1: Diabetes and Pregnancy: A Delicate Dance

Pregnancy is a time of joy and anticipation, but for women with diabetes, it can also be a time of increased vigilance and careful management. Imagine walking a tightrope while juggling—that's a bit like what it's like to navigate pregnancy with diabetes. You're constantly balancing blood sugar levels, medications, and potential complications, all while nurturing a growing life inside you.

Gestational Diabetes: A Temporary Guest with Lasting Impact

Gestational diabetes (GDM) is like an unexpected houseguest who shows up during pregnancy and can overstay their welcome. It's a form of diabetes that develops during pregnancy, even if you've never had it before. Think of it as your body's way of saying, "Hey, I'm a bit overwhelmed with all these hormonal changes, and I need some extra help managing blood sugar."

The good news is that GDM usually goes away after delivery, but it can increase your risk of developing type 2 diabetes later on. It's like a warning sign from your body, reminding you to prioritize your health.

Pre-existing Diabetes: A Familiar Companion on a New Journey

For women with pre-existing type 1 or type 2 diabetes, pregnancy is like embarking on a familiar hiking trail with a new twist. You know the terrain, but you also know that the added weight and changing conditions require extra caution.

Managing diabetes during pregnancy is like a delicate dance, requiring constant adjustments to your insulin regimen or other medications. It's like fine-tuning a musical instrument to ensure that every note is perfectly in tune.

The Stakes: Maternal and Fetal Health

The impact of diabetes on both mother and baby can be significant. Imagine a garden where the soil is either too dry or too wet—the plants won't thrive. Similarly, poorly controlled blood sugar levels can create an unfavorable environment for the developing baby.

For the mother, diabetes can increase the risk of complications like preeclampsia (a dangerous rise in blood pressure), cesarean delivery, and even future health problems like type 2 diabetes. It's like a ripple effect, with consequences that can extend far beyond pregnancy.

For the baby, diabetes can increase the risk of birth defects, excessive growth (macrosomia), and low blood sugar (hypoglycemia) after birth. It's like a recipe with too much or too little of a key ingredient—the outcome may not be what you expect.

A Case in Point: Sarah's Story

Sarah, a vibrant 32-year-old with type 1 diabetes, was overjoyed to discover she was pregnant. She had been managing her diabetes for years, but pregnancy threw her a curveball. Despite her best efforts, her blood sugar levels fluctuated, and she developed preeclampsia.

Sarah's story is a reminder that even with the best care and intentions, complications can arise. It's like a detour on a road trip—you may encounter unexpected obstacles, but you can still reach your destination with patience and perseverance.

Subtopic 2: Exercise: A Powerful Ally in Pregnancy with Diabetes

Exercise is like a magic potion for pregnant women with diabetes. It's a natural way to improve blood sugar control, reduce the risk of complications, boost cardiovascular health, and lift your spirits. Think of it as a superhero cape that empowers you to take charge of your health and your pregnancy.

Improved Glycemic Control: A Balancing Act

Exercise is like a tightrope walker's balancing pole, helping you maintain steady blood sugar levels. It increases insulin sensitivity, allowing your body to use glucose more effectively. It's like teaching your cells to become better listeners to insulin's instructions.

Reduced Risk of Complications: A Shield Against Adversity

Exercise is like a shield, protecting you from the potential complications of diabetes during pregnancy. It can lower your risk of preeclampsia, gestational hypertension, and even cardiovascular problems. It's like building a fortress around your body and your baby.

Enhanced Psychological Well-being: A Mood Booster

Exercise is like a dose of sunshine on a cloudy day, brightening your mood and reducing stress. It releases endorphins, natural mood boosters that can help you feel more positive and resilient. It's like a mental massage, easing away tension and promoting relaxation.

Safety First: A Cautious Approach

While exercise is generally safe and beneficial during pregnancy with diabetes, it's important to listen to your body and follow your healthcare provider's guidance. It's like embarking on a hike—you wouldn't set off without a map and proper gear.

A Case in Point: Maria's Triumph

Maria, a 28-year-old with gestational diabetes, was initially hesitant to exercise. But with her doctor's encouragement, she started with short walks and gradually increased her activity level. She also joined a prenatal yoga class, finding solace in the gentle movements and camaraderie.

Maria's story is a testament to the power of exercise in managing diabetes during pregnancy. It's like a dance of empowerment, allowing you to move with grace and strength through this transformative journey.

Conclusion: A Symphony of Care

Pregnancy with diabetes is like a symphony, with various instruments playing together to create a harmonious outcome. By combining meticulous blood sugar control, comprehensive prenatal care, and the power of exercise, women with diabetes can orchestrate a healthy pregnancy and a beautiful birth.

Future Directions: A Quest for Knowledge

Research continues to shed light on the intricacies of diabetes and pregnancy, paving the way for new strategies and interventions. It's like exploring uncharted territory, with each discovery bringing us closer to optimizing outcomes for mothers and babies.

The goal is to empower women with diabetes to embrace pregnancy with confidence and joy, knowing that they have the tools and support to navigate this extraordinary journey. It's like a beacon of hope, guiding us towards a future where diabetes and pregnancy can coexist in harmony.

Subtopic 3: Exercise Prescriptions and Safety Guidelines

Evidence-based recommendations for exercise type, intensity, duration, and frequency in pregnant women with diabetes, considering individual needs, risk factors, and stage of pregnancy.

Introduction

Pregnancy is a time of great joy and anticipation, but for women with diabetes, it can also be a time of increased vigilance and careful planning. Exercise, while beneficial for all expectant mothers, takes on a special significance for those with diabetes. It's a powerful tool for managing blood sugar, promoting overall health, and ensuring a smoother pregnancy journey. However, it's not a one-size-fits-all approach. This section delves into the evidence-based recommendations for exercise prescription in pregnant women with diabetes, emphasizing the importance of personalized plans that consider individual needs, risk factors, and the ever-changing landscape of pregnancy.

Benefits of Exercise in Pregnant Women with Diabetes

Imagine exercise as a gentle dance between you and your body, a dance that brings harmony to your blood sugar, strengthens your heart, and prepares you for the marathon of childbirth. For pregnant women with diabetes, this dance is even more crucial, offering a wealth of benefits:

Glycemic Control Maestro: Exercise acts as a conductor, orchestrating improved insulin sensitivity, leading to better blood sugar regulation and reducing the risk of hyperglycemia.

Weight Management Partner: Exercise helps you maintain a healthy weight gain during pregnancy, preventing complications associated with excessive weight gain.

Gestational Diabetes Guardian: For women with pre-existing diabetes, exercise can be a shield, helping to prevent the development of gestational diabetes.

Cardiovascular Champion: Exercise strengthens your heart and lungs, improving overall cardiovascular fitness.

Preeclampsia Preventer: Regular physical activity can lower the risk of preeclampsia, a serious pregnancy complication characterized by high blood pressure.

Mood Booster: Exercise releases endorphins, natural mood elevators that combat stress, anxiety, and depression, promoting emotional well-being during pregnancy.

Labor and Delivery Hero: Women who exercise regularly during pregnancy may experience shorter labor and fewer complications during delivery.

Exercise Prescription Considerations

Creating an exercise plan for pregnant women with diabetes is like crafting a bespoke suit – it needs to fit perfectly. Factors to consider include:

   Type of Diabetes: The type of diabetes (type 1, type 2, or gestational) influences exercise recommendations. Women with type 1 diabetes may require more frequent blood glucose monitoring and adjustments to insulin doses.
   Pre-pregnancy Fitness Level: Women who were physically active before pregnancy can generally maintain a higher level of exercise intensity. However, it's crucial to start gradually and listen to your body's whispers.
   Current Blood Glucose Control: Well-controlled blood sugar levels are the foundation for safe exercise. Women with unstable blood glucose should consult their healthcare provider before starting any exercise program.
   Presence of Complications: Certain pregnancy complications, such as preeclampsia or placenta previa, may require modifications to exercise routines.
   Stage of Pregnancy: Exercise recommendations evolve with each trimester, adapting to the physical changes and ensuring safety.

Exercise Type

A variety of exercises can be woven into your pregnancy routine, offering a tapestry of benefits:

   Aerobic Exercise: Brisk walking, swimming, cycling, and low-impact aerobics are excellent choices. Aim for at least 30 minutes of moderate-intensity aerobic exercise most days of the week.
   Strength Training: Strength training exercises using light weights or resistance bands can help maintain muscle

mass and strength. Focus on exercises that target major muscle groups, such as squats, lunges, and bicep curls.

Flexibility Exercises: Stretching and yoga can improve flexibility, reduce muscle tension, and promote relaxation.

Exercise Intensity

Exercise intensity should be moderate, allowing for comfortable conversation during the activity. The "talk test" is a simple way to gauge intensity. If you can talk comfortably while exercising, you're likely at a moderate intensity. If you're too breathless to talk, you may be exercising too intensely.

Exercise Duration and Frequency

Aim for at least 30 minutes of moderate-intensity exercise most days of the week. If you're new to exercise, start with shorter sessions and gradually increase the duration as your fitness improves.

Exercise Safety Guidelines

Consult Your Healthcare Provider: Before starting any exercise program, discuss your plans with your healthcare provider. They can assess your individual needs and provide personalized recommendations.

Monitor Blood Glucose Levels: Check your blood glucose levels before, during, and after exercise, especially if you have type 1 diabetes.

Stay Hydrated: Drink plenty of water before, during, and after exercise to prevent dehydration.

Avoid Overheating: Exercise in a cool environment and wear loose-fitting, breathable clothing.

Listen to Your Body: Pay attention to your body's signals and stop if you experience any pain, discomfort, or dizziness.

Avoid High-Impact Activities: Activities that involve jumping or jarring motions can put stress on your joints and may increase the risk of injury.

Modify Exercises as Needed: As your pregnancy progresses, you may need to modify exercises to accommodate physical changes. For example, you may need to switch from high-impact activities to low-impact options.

Case Study

Maria, a 32-year-old woman with type 1 diabetes, was overjoyed to discover she was pregnant. Having managed her diabetes with insulin and a healthy diet, she was determined to continue exercising during her pregnancy. Maria consulted her healthcare provider, who recommended a moderate-intensity exercise program consisting of brisk walking, swimming, and prenatal yoga. Maria started with 20-minute sessions three times a week and gradually increased the duration and frequency as her pregnancy progressed. She diligently monitored her blood glucose levels and adjusted her insulin doses as needed. Throughout her pregnancy, Maria experienced excellent glycemic control, maintained a healthy weight gain, and had a smooth labor and delivery.

Conclusion

Exercise is an integral part of prenatal care for women with diabetes. By following evidence-based recommendations and working closely with their healthcare providers, women with diabetes can safely engage in physical activity throughout their pregnancy, reaping the numerous benefits for both themselves and their babies.

Subtopic 4: Multidisciplinary Care for Optimal Outcomes

Emphasis on the importance of collaborative care between obstetricians, endocrinologists, and exercise specialists to optimize maternal and fetal health in diabetes, ensuring safe and effective exercise participation throughout pregnancy.

Introduction

Managing diabetes during pregnancy is like navigating a complex maze, requiring a team of experts to guide you through each twist and turn. Collaborative care between obstetricians, endocrinologists, and exercise specialists is the compass that ensures optimal maternal and fetal health. This section highlights the importance of interdisciplinary collaboration in prenatal care, patient education, and exercise prescription, creating a safety net for expectant mothers with diabetes.

The Multidisciplinary Team

The multidisciplinary team involved in the care of pregnant women with diabetes is like an orchestra, each member playing a vital role in creating a harmonious symphony of care:

   Obstetrician: The obstetrician is the conductor, providing prenatal care, monitoring the pregnancy, and managing any pregnancy-related complications.
   Endocrinologist: The endocrinologist is the diabetes specialist, fine-tuning blood glucose levels during pregnancy.
   Exercise Specialist: The exercise specialist is the choreographer, designing a safe and effective exercise program tailored to the individual needs and stage of pregnancy.

Registered Dietitian: The registered dietitian is the nutritionist, providing guidance on healthy eating habits and creating a meal plan that supports both diabetes management and pregnancy needs.

Diabetes Educator: The diabetes educator is the coach, providing education and support on diabetes self-management, including blood glucose monitoring, medication management, and healthy lifestyle choices.

Importance of Collaborative Care

Collaborative care ensures that pregnant women with diabetes receive comprehensive and coordinated care from a team of experts. Each member of the team brings unique knowledge and skills to the table, contributing to a holistic approach to diabetes management during pregnancy.

Benefits of Collaborative Care

Improved Glycemic Control: Close collaboration between the endocrinologist and obstetrician ensures that blood glucose levels are closely monitored and managed throughout pregnancy.

Reduced Risk of Complications: Early detection and management of pregnancy complications, such as preeclampsia or preterm labor, are enhanced through collaborative care.

Optimized Exercise Prescription: The exercise specialist works closely with the obstetrician and endocrinologist to develop an exercise program that is safe and effective for the individual woman's needs and stage of pregnancy.

Enhanced Patient Education: The multidisciplinary team provides comprehensive education on diabetes management, pregnancy care, and healthy lifestyle choices.

Improved Patient Satisfaction: Women who receive collaborative care report higher levels of satisfaction with their prenatal care experience.

Prenatal Care

Prenatal care for women with diabetes involves regular check-ups with the obstetrician and endocrinologist. These visits include:

Blood Glucose Monitoring: Regular blood glucose checks are essential to assess glycemic control and make adjustments to medication or insulin doses as needed.
Weight Management: Monitoring weight gain during pregnancy helps ensure a healthy pregnancy and reduce the risk of complications.
Blood Pressure Monitoring: Regular blood pressure checks help detect and manage preeclampsia, a serious pregnancy complication.
Fetal Monitoring: Ultrasounds and other fetal monitoring techniques are used to assess the baby's growth and development.

Patient Education

Patient education is a crucial component of multidisciplinary care. The team provides education on:

Diabetes Management: Self-monitoring of blood glucose, medication management, and healthy eating habits.
Exercise Guidelines: Safe and effective exercise recommendations for pregnancy.
Pregnancy Care: Information on prenatal care, labor and delivery, and postpartum care.
Warning Signs: Recognizing and responding to potential complications.

Case Study

Sarah, a 28-year-old woman with gestational diabetes, was referred to a multidisciplinary team for prenatal care. The team consisted of an obstetrician, endocrinologist, exercise specialist, and registered dietitian. Sarah received regular check-ups with the obstetrician and endocrinologist, who closely monitored her blood glucose levels and made adjustments to her meal plan as needed. The exercise specialist developed a personalized exercise program for Sarah, consisting of walking, swimming, and prenatal yoga. The registered dietitian provided guidance on healthy eating habits and helped Sarah create a meal plan that met her nutritional needs and managed her blood glucose levels. Throughout her pregnancy, Sarah benefited from the collaborative care of the multidisciplinary team. She maintained excellent glycemic control, had a healthy pregnancy, and delivered a healthy baby.

Conclusion

Multidisciplinary care is the cornerstone of optimal maternal and fetal health in pregnant women with diabetes. Collaborative care between obstetricians, endocrinologists, exercise specialists, and other healthcare professionals ensures comprehensive support, guidance, and education throughout pregnancy. By working together, the team can empower women with diabetes to achieve a healthy pregnancy and deliver healthy babies.

About Author

Dr. Azhar ul Haque Sario is a bestselling author and data scientist with a remarkable record of achievement. This Cambridge alumnus brings a wealth of knowledge to his work, holding an MBA, ACCA (Knowledge Level - FTMS College Malaysia), BBA, and several Google certifications, including specializations in Google Data Analytics, Google Digital Marketing & E-commerce, and Google Project Management.

With ten years of business experience, Azhar combines practical expertise with his impressive academic background to craft insightful books. His prolific writing has resulted in an astounding 2810 published titles, earning him the record for the maximum Kindle editions and paperback books published by an individual author in one year, awarded by Asia Books of Records in 2024. This extraordinary achievement has also led to Azhar being awarded an honorary PhD from World Records University UK, which he will soon receive.

ORCID: https://orcid.org/0009-0004-8629-830X
Azhar.sario@hotmail.co.uk
https://www.linkedin.com/in/azharulhaquesario/

www.ingramcontent.com/pod-product-compliance
Ingram Content Group UK Ltd.
Pitfield, Milton Keynes, MK11 3LW, UK
UKHW030025120225
454951UK00004B/277